The Classic
QUIZ
BOOK 1

Edited by ROBIN DYNES

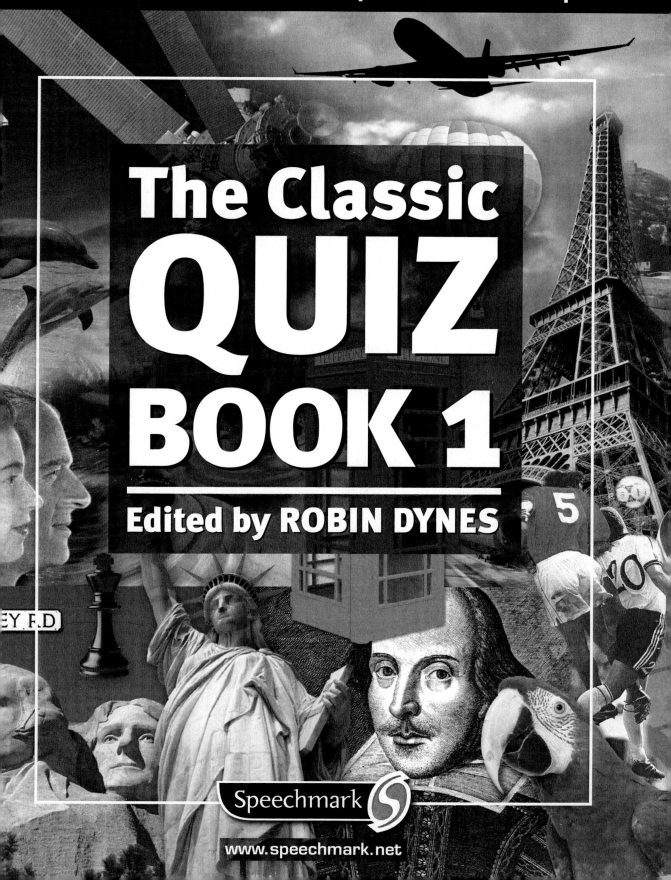

The Classic
QUIZ
BOOK 1

Edited by ROBIN DYNES

Speechmark

www.speechmark.net

Published by
Speechmark Publishing Ltd, Sunningdale House, 43 Caldecotte Lake Drive, Milton Keynes MK7 8LF,
United Kingdom
Tel: +44 (0)1908 277177   Fax: +44 (0)1908 278297
www.speechmark.net

002-4168/Printed in the United Kingdom by CMP (UK) Ltd

British Library Cataloguing in Publication Data
A catalogue record for this book is available from
the British Library

ISBN 978 0 86388 440 5

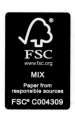

Contents

This quiz book has been designed and prepared specifically for use with therapeutic groups. The main considerations have been as follows:

- To provide an adult quiz book with questions which are realistically within the scope of the average person;
- To provide a wide variety of interesting and stimulating topics;
- To provide the facility for patients or clients to choose their own topics;
- To enable the group leader to locate the required topic rapidly;
- To supply questions in each section at three levels of difficulty so that the leader can select a question to suit the patient's or client's ability;
- To position answers adjacent to each question for the leader's convenience.

HOW TO USE THIS BOOK

There are 50 sections divided into 40 specific and 10 general knowledge topics.

The questions for each topic lie in a double page spread and in most cases are divided thus:

LEVEL A — 10 easy questions

LEVEL B — 20 questions of medium difficulty

LEVEL C — 10 hard questions

Sport

LEVEL A

1 With which sport is Wimbledon associated? . . . . . **Tennis** ✓
2 With which sport do you associate Jack Nicklaus? . . . **Golf**
3 Which boxer called himself 'the greatest'? . . . . . **Muhammad Ali** ✓
4 John MacEnroe became famous in which sport? . . . . **Tennis**
5 How many players are there in a cricket team? . . . . **11** ✓
6 How often are the summer Olympic Games held? . . . **Every 4 years**
7 In basketball, how many points are scored each time a player shoots the ball into the basket? **2**
8 What does a caddy do? . . . . **Carries golf clubs** ✓
9 How many players are there on each side in a game of football? . **11** ✓
10 With what two items do you play badminton? . . . . . **A racket and a shuttlecock**

LEVEL B

1 What do the symbols on the Olympic flag represent? . . . **The five continents of the world**
2 In which sport did Olga Korbut excel? . . . . . . **Gymnastics**
3 Who was the first man to run a mile in less than 4 minutes? . . **Roger Bannister**
4 How many players are there in a rugby union side? . . . **15**
5 What is the name given to a score of 40–40 in tennis? . . . **Deuce**
6 In golf, what 'under par' is an eagle? **2**
7 The America's Cup, originally presented in 1851, is a trophy for which sport? . . . . **Yachting**
8 On a dart board, what is the highest you can score with three darts? **180**
9 Name the swimmer who won 7 gold medals in the 1972 Olympic games . . . . **Mark Spitz**
10 In show jumping, how many faults for a refusal? **3**

11 How many holes are there on a full size golf course? **18**

12 Which athletic events all take place from circles? . . . . **Shot-put, discus and hammer**

13 With which sport do you associate Mario Andretti? . . . . **Motor racing**

14 Name the five colours of an archery target. . . . . . **Gold, red, blue, black and white**

15 Who was the athlete who won 4 gold medals in the 1936 Berlin Olympic Games? . . . . **Jesse Owens**

16 What boxing weight class falls between bantam-weight and light-weight? . . . . **Feather-weight**

17 In which sport would you use the term face-off? . . . . **Ice hockey**

18 Batting, fielding and pitching are skills used in which sport? . **Baseball**

19 How many miles are run in a marathon? **26**

20 What is a period of play in polo known as? . . . . . . **A chukka**

LEVEL C

1 Where were the 1960 Olympics held? . . . . **Rome**

2 In what sport did Wilma Rudolph achieve fame? . . . . **Sprinting**

3 Lacrosse, basketball and five-pin bowling all originated from which country? . . . . **Canada**

4 In which sport are the terms single axle, triple salko and butterfly used? . . . . **Ice figure skating**

5 Who was the 'Brown Bomber'? . . . . **Joe Louis**

6 What is the more common name by which the popular world-wide sport Toxophily is known? . . . . . . **Archery**

7 Which is older, the London or the New York marathon? . . . **New York**

8 Before Bjorn Borg, who won Wimbledon in three consecutive years? **Fred Perry**

9 What is the meaning of the word 'Karate'? . . . . . . **Empty hand**

10 The squat, bench press and deadlift are terms used in what sport? **Powerlifting**

Popular Music

LEVEL A

1 With which musical instrument do you associate the musician Larry Adler? . . . . **Harmonica (mouth organ)**

2 Which singer lived at *Gracelands*? . . . . **Elvis Presley**

3 By which nickname was Louis Armstrong known? . . . **Satchmo**

4 What were 'sweeter than wine' according to the Beatles? . . **Kisses**

5 What was Glen Miller's signature tune? . . . . . . *Moonlight Serenade*

6 Which city is known as the home of jazz? . . . . . . *New Orleans*

7 From which musical did the hit *Don't Cry For Me Argentina* come? .*Evita*

8 In the song, how many trombones were there? **76**

9 Which collaborators wrote the music and lyrics for *South Pacific*? **Rodgers & Hammerstein**

10 How did Buddy Holly die? . . . . **In an air crash**

LEVEL B

1 Who played the part of Eliza Doolittle in the musical film *My Fair Lady*? . . . . **Audrey Hepburn**

2 Who sang *Falling In Love Again* in the film *Blue Angel*? . . . **Marlene Dietrich**

3 Who made the best selling album *Thriller*? . . . . . **Michael Jackson**

4 Who sang the hit *In My Heart and In My Soul*? . . . . **Rod Stewart**

5 In which country did reggae originate? . . . . . . **Jamaica**

6 What instrument does jazzman Stephane Grappelli play? . . **Violin**

7 How many hours away from Tulsa was Gene Pitney? **24**

8 Who wrote the song *Smoke Gets In Your Eyes*? . . . . . **Jerome Kern**

9 From which musical does the song *There's No Business Like Showbusiness* come? . . . . *Annie Get Your Gun*

10 Who won an Oscar for her part in the film *Mary Poppins*? . . **Julie Andrews**

11 Which singer left the Supremes to become a superstar
    solo performer? . . . . **Diana Ross**

12 *Love Me Do* was the first hit record for which group? . . . **The Beatles**

13 To which tune is *The Battle Hymn of the Republic* sung? . . . ***John Brown's Body***

14 Which song did Rick ask Sam to play in the film *Casablanca?* . ***As Time Goes By***

15 *Bridge Over Troubled Water* was a hit for which duo? . . . **Simon and Garfunkel**

16 *Lady Sings The Blues* is whose life story? . . . . . **Billie Holiday**

17 Which group's first hit was *It's All Over Now?* . . . . . **The Rolling Stones**

18 What musical told us to 'keep talking happy talk'? . . . . ***South Pacific***

19 For what is a platinum record awarded? . . . . . . **An LP selling a million
                                                          records**

20 Who sang about *The Good Ship Lollipop* in the 1934 film
    Bright Eyes? . . . . **Shirley Temple**

LEVEL C

1 Who sang about *Your Cheatin' Heart?* . . . . . . **Hank Williams**

2 Name the rival gangs in the film *West Side Story*. . . . . **Jets and Sharks**

3 *Thanks For The Memory* was the theme tune for which comedian? **Bob Hope**

4 Which singer was the subject of the film *Lonely Boy?* . . . **Paul Anka**

5 Who sang *The Legend of Cat Ballou* in the 1965 film *Cat Ballou?* **Nat King Cole**

6 Who sang about *Summer Nights?* . . . . **John Travolta &
                                                     Olivia Newton John**

7 In which film did Doris Day sing the song *Secret Love?* . . . ***Calamity Jane***

8 From which Andrew Lloyd-Webber musical does the hit song
   Any Dream Will Do come? . . . . ***Joseph and his Amazing
                                                    Technicolour Dreamcoat***

9 Which star, known for his country music, wrote the all-time
   favourite *Country Roads?* . . . . **John Denver**

10 Which French singer was associated with a straw hat
    and the film *Gigi?* . . . . **Maurice Chevalier**

LEVEL A

1	The type of vacation that newly-weds go on.	**Honeymoon**
2	A place where you can borrow books.	**Library**
3	Covering for hand with separate divisions for fingers.	**Glove**
4	Place or hall in which justice is administered.	**Court**
5	Small piece of steel used in sewing with a thread.	**Needle**
6	A building for public Christian worship.	**Church**
7	The season in which vegetation begins to appear.	**Spring**
8	Toy that you fly on a long piece of string.	**Kite**
9	Place where milk and its products are processed or sold.	**Dairy**
10	A place where you would buy meat.	**Butcher's shop**

LEVEL B

1	A person who teaches dance steps and routines.	**Choreographer**
2	A puppet worked by strings.	**Marionette**
3	A person who specializes in tracing family descent.	**Genealogist**
4	Young male horse.	**Colt**
5	Solidified lava used for rubbing stains from the skin.	**Pumice stone**
6	Thread made from animal intestines used for rackets and musical instruments.	**Gut**
7	Brown oily liquid distilled from coal tar.	**Creosote**
8	A long narrow sledge curved upwards at the front used for going downhill over snow.	**Toboggan**
9	Mass or river of ice moving very slowly.	**Glacier**
10	Small shop selling fashionable clothes.	**Boutique**

11	An event regarded as a prophetic sign.	Omen
12	A person who deals in fur or fur clothes.	Furrier
13	Bar of iron with a bent end used as a lever.	Crowbar
14	Person who rakes in stakes and pays out winnings at a gaming table.	Croupier
15	Pin thrust through meat to hold it compactly in cooking.	Skewer
16	A sum of money or article bequeathed by a predecessor.	Legacy
17	Large man-like animal said to exist in the Himalayas	Yeti (Abominable Snowman)
18	The chest muscles.	Pectorals
19	A male bird with tail-coverts that can be expanded erect like a fan in a splendid colourful display.	Peacock
20	Woman's small private room.	Boudoir

LEVEL C

1	A person in his or her eighties.	Octogenarian
2	A doctor who studies and treats mental disorders.	Psychiatrist
3	Turkish tobacco-pipe with a long tube passing through water.	Hookah
4	Frame with balls sliding on rods used for counting.	Abacus
5	A tendency for self-worship.	Narcissism
6	To dig up a buried corpse.	To exhume
7	Food that cattle bring back from the stomach and chew again.	Cud
8	Using four transmission channels.	Quadraphonic
9	An artist's slab (often wooden) held in the hand and used for holding and mixing colours when painting.	Palette
10	The study of the characteristics of handwriting.	Graphology

Air & Water

LEVEL A

1. Pellets of frozen rain. . . . . **Hail**
2. What do we call the massive pieces of ice which break loose from the polar caps? . . . . **Icebergs**
3. What distinguishes sea water from fresh water? . . . . **Salt in the sea water**
4. What type of ship carries oil in bulk? . . . . . . **Tanker**
5. Name the aircraft which flies with no power except the wind. . **Glider**
6. What is the look-out platform on the mast of a ship called? . **Crow's nest**
7. What does maritime mean? . . . . **Concerning the sea**
8. What is the name of the wet field that rice is grown in? . . **Paddy field**
9. What is a reservoir? . . . . **A natural or artificial lake that is a source or store of water**
10. Which large passenger ship sank on her maiden voyage? . . *Titanic*

LEVEL B

1. Which is the largest ocean on the Earth's surface? . . . **Pacific**
2. In which year was the Suez Canal opened? **1869**
3. Which famous city is sinking? . . . . **Venice**
4. What is a natural fountain of water called? . . . . . **Geyser**
5. What are the two main gaseous substances in the air? . . **Oxygen and nitrogen**
6. In 1872 a ship was found abandoned in the Atlantic with no signs of life. What was its name? . . . . *Marie Celeste*
7. What do scientists call the class of creatures to which shrimps, lobsters and crab belong? . . . . **Crustaceans**
8. What is the rainy season in South Asia called? . . . . **Monsoon**
9. Which famous artist designed 'flying machines'? . . . **Leonardo da Vinci**
10. What is an amphibious aircraft? . . . . **One that can land and take off from either land or water**

11	Scientists who study the sea, its depth etc, are known as what?	**Oceanographers**
12	What is an explosive underwater missile called?	**Torpedo**
13	What are the bowl-shaped holes on the moon called? . . .	**Craters**
14	How many arms has a star fish?	**5**
15	Approximately what percentage of the Earth's surface is covered by water?	**75%**
16	Which liner lies half submerged in the Bay of Hong Kong? . .	***Queen Elizabeth I***
17	What is a Portuguese man-of-war?	**Jelly-fish**
18	What is the name of the drifting mass of life made up of billions of minute living creatures in the sea?	**Plankton**
19	How does heat reach us from the sun?	**Radiation**
20	What is significant about the *Enola Gay*?	**American aircraft which dropped the first atomic bomb**

LEVEL C

1	What is the nearest galaxy to our own?	**Andromeda**
2	What does a hygrometer measure?	**Humidity**
3	What is so unusual about water when it freezes? . . .	**It is the only liquid that expands when frozen**
4	In which year was the first joint Russian-American mission in space?	**1975**
5	Where would you find a nimbostratus?	**In the sky – it is a cloud**
6	Name the 5 climatic zones of the Earth	**2 polar, 2 temperate, 1 tropical**
7	Who did the ancient Greeks believe threw down lightning bolts during thunderstorms?	**Zeus**
8	Which is the most prevalent gas in the air?	**Nitrogen**
9	How many moons has Mars?	**2**
10	Why would an astronaut have to crawl on the planet Jupiter? .	**The astronaut would weigh much more due to the strong gravity pull**

All to do with Numbers

LEVEL A

1	How many years in a decade?	10
2	What does 'tri' mean at the beginning of a word?	3
3	How many in a dozen?	12
4	How many seasons are there?	4
5	How many pints in a gallon?	8
6	How many eyes did the Cyclops have?	1
7	How many lives is a cat said to have?	9
8	How many years does it take the Earth to travel once round the sun?	1
9	How many sides has a cube?	6
10	How many arms or tentacles has an octopus?	8

LEVEL B

1	How many in a baker's dozen?	13
2	What is a thousand thousands?	**One million**
3	How many wonders of the world were there?	7
4	What is the square root of 169?	13
5	How many pockets has a snooker table?	6
6	How many stars and stripes are there in the American flag?	**13 red and white stripes, 50 stars**
7	How many pieces are there on a chessboard?	32
8	How many days in a leap year?	366
9	How many Psalms are there in the book of Psalms?	150
10	What is the square of 8?	64

11	How many lines has a limerick?	5
12	How many days in October?	31
13	How many books are there in the *New Testament*? . . .	27
14	How many coloured squares has a Rubik Cube?	54
15	What value is Pi as a fraction?	22/7
16	How many in a gross?	144
17	How many is a score?	20
18	How many dalmations are there in the children's book which was made into a film by Walt Disney?	101
19	In Casco Bay, Maine, USA there are a number of islands whose name gives away their number. How many are there? . . .	365 (Calendar Islands)
20	How many lines has a sonnet?	14

LEVEL C

1	How many symphonies did Beethoven write?	9
2	How many days did the famous Long March of the Chinese Communists (1934–35) last?	368 days
3	When did the American Revolutionary War break out? . . .	1775
4	How many cards in a tarot pack?	78
5	What is the atomic number of gold?	79
6	According to the poem by Tennyson, how many horsemen took part in the Charge of the Light Brigade?	600
7	What is 17 squared?	289
8	In which year was the first supersonic airliner flown? . . .	1968
9	What is the value of the Roman numerals CCLVI?	256
10	How many muses were there?	9

Inventions & Discoveries

LEVEL A

1 What did Louis Braille invent? . . . . **A dot alphabet for the blind**

2 Which continent did Christopher Columbus discover? . . . **America**

3 What did John Dunlop invent? . . . . **Air filled rubber tyre**

4 Who discovered that germs could be killed by heat and first introduced pasteurised milk? . . . . **Louis Pasteur**

5 Which scientist do you associate with an apple? . . . . . **Isaac Newton**

6 What did Isaac Pitman invent? . . . . **Shorthand**

7 Alexander Graham Bell invented a communication instrument. What was it? . . . . **Telephone**

8 Which famous American car manufacturer built his first car in 1896? **Henry Ford**

9 Which explorer brought potatoes to Britain? . . . . . . **Sir Walter Raleigh**

10 What was the surname of Orville and Wilbur who flew the first aeroplane? . . . . **Wright**

LEVEL B

1 What was the name of the first communication satellite in orbit with the earth? It became a global courier of TV programmes in 1965. . . . . *Early Bird*

2 Which famous naturalist wrote *The Origin of Species*? . . . **Charles Darwin**

3 Who was the American explorer who was the first person to fly over both the North and South Poles and across the Atlantic Ocean? . . . . **Richard Evelyn Byrd**

4 'Sound Navigation and Ranging System' was a technique for generating sound waves of a very high frequency to detect sub-marine objects that was perfected in the Second World War. By what name was it better known? . . . . **Sonar**

5 Which American invented the Kodak camera in 1888? . . . **George Eastman**

6 Which German invented the mercury thermometer in 1714? . . **Gabriel Fahrenheit**

7 Who invented the light bulb? . . . . **Thomas Edison**

8 Tasman discovered Van Dieman's Land but what was this renamed? . . . . **Tasmania**

9 Who was the American inventor of the magnetic telegraph? . . **Samuel Morse**

10 Who put forward the theory of relativity? . . . . . . **Einstein**

11 Which famous woman discovered radium and plutonium? . . **Marie Curie**

12 What did Cecil Booth invent which helps to keep the house clean? **Vacuum cleaner**

13 Which Frenchman, in 1942, assisted in the design and development of the aqualung? . . . . **Jacques Cousteau**

14 What did Marconi invent? . . . . **Radio**

15 Which American invented vulcanized rubber? . . . . **Charles Goodyear**

16 Who was the founder of the international communist movement? **Karl Marx**

17 Who was the Greek scientist who invented a device to raise water from one level to another? . . . . **Archimedes**

18 Name the zeppelin which caught fire and exploded in 1937. . . **Hindenburg**

19 Who was the first man to orbit the Earth in space? . . . . **Yuri Gagarin**

20 Which American invented the frozen food process in 1925? . . **Clarence Birdseye**

LEVEL C

1 The Spanish explorer Fernando de Soto discovered which famous American river? . . . . **The Mississippi**

2 Who invented the bunsen burner? . . . . **Robert Wilhelm Bunsen**

3 Which Swedish chemist invented dynamite? . . . . . . **Alfred Nobel**

4 Who invented the wind-scale? . . . . **Admiral Beaufort**

5 What were the first words recorded by Thomas Edison when he made the first recording of sound on 6 December 1877? . . . **'Mary had a little lamb'**

6 Who invented the safety razor in 1895? . . . . . . **King C Gillette**

7 Who discovered Greenland? . . . . **Eric the Red**

8 Which American statesman invented the lightning conductor? . **Benjamin Franklin**

9 Who invented the revolver? . . . . **Samuel Colt**

10 What did the Italian Galileo Galilei invent in the 1590s which is still used today? . . . . **The thermometer**

Homes

LEVEL A

Where do the following live?

1	Mouse	**Hole, nest**
2	Dog	**Kennel**
3	Bird	**Nest**
4	Car	**Garage**
5	Spider	**Web**
6	Nun	**Convent**
7	Native American	**Wigwam, tepee**
8	Eskimo	**Igloo**
9	King	**Palace, Castle**
10	Books	**Library**

LEVEL B

1	Snail	**Shell**
2	Soldier	**Barracks, camp**
3	Sailor	**Ship**
4	The Pope	**The Vatican**
5	Gypsy	**Caravan**
6	Convict	**Prison**
7	Monk	**Monastry**
8	Horse	**Stable**
9	Sheep	**Pen, fold**
10	Aeroplane	**Hangar**

11	Vicar	. . . .	**Vicarage**
12	Bee	. . . .	**Hive**
13	Wine	. . . .	**Cellar**
14	US President	. . . .	**White House**
15	Pig	. . . .	**Sty**
16	Peas	. . . .	**Pod**
17	British Prime Minister	. . . .	**10 Downing Street**
18	Chicken	. . . .	**Coop**
19	Guns	. . . .	**Armoury**
20	Lumberjack	. . . .	**Log cabin**

LEVEL C

1	Eagle	. . . .	**Eyrie**
2	Pigeon	. . . .	**Dove cote**
3	Tortoise	. . . .	**Shell**
4	Ape	. . . .	**Tree, nest**
5	Wasp	. . . .	**Nest, vespiary**
6	Grain	. . . .	**Granary**
7	Parson	. . . .	**Parsonage**
8	Minister	. . . .	**Manse**
9	Squirrel	. . . .	**Drey**
10	Rabbit	. . . .	**Warren, burrow**

Do-it-Yourself

LEVEL A

1 What does a plane do? . . . . Smooths wooden surfaces
2 Why would you insulate pipes supplying water in the household? . . . . To stop the water freezing during cold weather
3 What is a brick trowel used for? . . . . . For placing mortar when laying bricks or concrete blocks
4 Apart from brushes, what other tool could be used to apply paint to walls? . . . . . Roller
5 How would you clean your brush after using a solvent (oil) based paint? . . . . . . With white spirit or turpentine
6 How would you clean your brush after using a water-based paint? . . . . With water
7 Where would you find a fuse? . . . . . . In an electric plug or fuse box
8 How would you know woodworm had infested a piece of wood? . . . . Small holes would appear in it
9 Where would you find rafters? . . . . . In the roof
10 Why would you insulate a hot water tank? . . To save energy by retaining heat in the tank

LEVEL B

1 What instrument is needed to check that shelves are perfectly horizontal? . . . . . . Spirit level
2 What is a plumb line? . . . . Any small but heavy weight hung on a length of string used for judging verticality
3 What are the basic substances which are mixed together to make mortar? . . . . . . Sand, cement and water
4 What should you do before working on anything that is operated by electricity? . . . . Turn off the supply of electricity
5 What is a stopcock? . . . . A tap which cuts off the supply of water
6 If a tap is dripping when it is turned off, what will need replacing? . . . . Washer
7 What would you be doing if you were using a coping saw? . . . . Cutting curves in wood
8 Apart from hammering nails in, what might you use a claw hammer for? . . . . Pulling nails out
9 Is oak a hard or a soft wood? . . . . . . Hard

10 What are cold chisels made from? . . . . . **Steel**

11 Cork, cushion, vinyl and parquet are all types of what? **Floor coverings**

12 What would you use creosote for? . . . . **Preserving outdoor timber**

13 Should a woodwork plane be stored with the sole down or on its side? . . . . . . **On its side**

14 What would you use solder for? . . . . **Joining metals**

15 Why would you bleed a radiator? . . . . . **To get rid of an air pocket which is stopping the circulation of water**

16 Where would you expect to find a float valve? . **In a water storage tank or toilet cistern**

17 What is a mitre joint used for? . . . . . **Joining the corner of frames**

18 What are switches that turn off when overloaded by current called? . . . . **Circuit breakers**

19 Where would you put coving? . . . . . **Between wall and ceiling**

20 What would you use bending springs for? . . **Bending pipes**

LEVEL C

1 What is the general direction of wood fibres known as? . . . . **Grain**

2 What does 'short circuit' mean? . . . . **The accidental re-routing of electricity to earth which increases the flow of current and blows a fuse**

3 What would you use to provide a hardcore to form a sub-base below pavings etc? . . . . **Broken bricks or stones**

4 What is an architrave? . . . . **The moulding around a door or window**

5 Is softwood usually cut from coniferous or deciduous trees? . . . . **Coniferous**

6 What is the term for applying a paste to a porous surface before hanging wallpaper? . . . . **Sizing or priming**

7 If a metal object has oxidized what has happened to it? . . . . **It has rusted**

8 Rasp cut, double cut and dreadnought are all types of what? . . . . **Files**

9 What problem would you have if you encountered a spreading mass of mycelium? . . . . . **Dry rot**

10 If something has been 'galvanized', what has happened to it? . . . . **It has been covered with a protective coating of zinc**

Famous Men

LEVEL A

1 Who was discovered in the cellars of the House of Lords in 1605 and was intending to blow it up with gunpowder? **Guy Fawkes**

2 Who became known as 'Ole blue eyes'? **Frank Sinatra**

3 Which famous king had a round table? **Arthur**

4 Which famous man in the Bible led the Israelites out of Egypt? **Moses**

5 Name the Beatles. **John Lennon, Ringo Starr, Paul McCartney, George Harrison**

6 What were Laurel and Hardy's first names? **Stan and Oliver**

7 Who was Queen Victoria's husband? **Prince Albert**

8 Who led the English at the Battle of Agincourt? **King Henry V**

9 Which famous dancer and actor was teamed with Ginger Rogers in *Top Hat* and many other films? **Fred Astaire**

10 Who was the famous British admiral who died in the Battle of Trafalgar? **Nelson**

LEVEL B

1 Who wrote *David Copperfield*? **Charles Dickens**

2 Name the composer of the *Messiah*. **Handel**

3 Who composed *White Christmas*, *Easter Parade* and more than 1,000 other popular songs? **Irving Berlin**

4 One of whose famous speeches ended 'We shall never surrender'? **Winston Churchill**

5 Who captained the *Golden Hind*? **Sir Francis Drake**

6 Which cartoon animator and film producer created Mickey Mouse? **Walt Disney**

7 Name the Marx brothers. **Zeppo, Groucho, Harpo and Chico**

8 Who was the President of the US who resigned during the Watergate investigation? **Richard Nixon**

9   Who wrote *The Great Gatsby* and *Tender is the Night*?   .   .   . **F Scott Fitzgerald**

10 Who was known as the 'King of Rock'?   .   .   .   .   .   . **Elvis Presley**

11 What did Jack Nicklaus do to become famous?   .   .   .   . **Played golf**

12 Who betrayed Jesus?   .   .   .   . **Judas Iscariot**

13 Which Olympic swimming champion became famous for his
    portrayal of Tarzan in 19 films?   .   .   .   . **Johnny Weissmuller**

14 Whose catchphrase was 'Play it again Sam'?   .   .   .   . **Humphrey Bogart**

15 Which Vice-President became President of the US after
    John F Kennedy was assassinated?   .   .   .   .   .   . **Lyndon B Johnson**

16 Who was the first man to step on the moon?   .   .   .   . **Neil Armstrong**

17 Which famous Roman dictator was stabbed by Brutus in 44BC?   . **Julius Caesar**

18 For what did Sigmund Freud achieve fame?   .   .   .   .   . **Psychoanalysis**

19 For what did Thomas Gainsborough achieve fame?   .   .   . **Painting**

20 Who became King of England in 1066?   .   .   .   .   .   . **William the Conqueror**

LEVEL C

1   Which South African surgeon performed the first heart transplant
    in 1967?   .   .   .   . **Christiaan Barnard**

2   In which city was Marco Polo born?   .   .   .   .   .   . **Venice**

3   Which French novelist is best known for his eight-volume work
    Remembrance of Things Past?   .   .   .   . **Marcel Proust**

4   Who shouted 'Eureka'?   .   .   .   . **Archimedes**

5   Which famous archbishop was murdered in Canterbury Cathedral? **Sir Thomas à Becket**

6   Which man was responsible for the first atomic bomb?   .   . **R J Oppenheimer**

7   Name the English founder of Methodism.   .   .   .   .   . **John Wesley**

8   Who wrote the music for *West Side Story*?   .   .   .   .   . **Leonard Bernstein**

9   Who made the speech 'Government of the people, by the people,
    for the people shall not perish from the earth'?   .   .   .   . **Abraham Lincoln**

10 Which short story writer and novelist created the private detective
    Philip Marlowe?   .   .   .   . **Raymond Chandler**

Famous Women

LEVEL A

1 Name the first woman British Prime Minister. . . . . . **Margaret Thatcher**
2 In which sport did Martina Navratilova become famous? . . **Tennis**
3 Who is Popeye's girlfriend? . . . . **Olive Oyl**
4 Which French peasant girl was burnt at the stake? . . . **Joan of Arc**
5 Who was the first woman created? . . . . **Eve**
6 Which famous actress's catchphrase was 'Come up and see me sometime'? . . . . **Mae West**
7 Who was Samson in love with? . . . . **Delilah**
8 How did Marie Tussaud achieve fame? . . . . . . **She founded the famous waxworks museum**
9 Of which country is Sophia Loren a native? . . . . . **Italy**
10 Why was Mrs Ghandhi famous? . . . . **She became Prime Minister of India**

LEVEL B

1 Who was Liza Minnelli's mother? . . . . **Judy Garland**
2 Which actress played Scarlet O'Hara in the film *Gone With The Wind*? . . . . **Vivien Leigh**
3 Name the queen of France guillotined in 1793. . . . . **Marie Antoinette**
4 For what was Maria Callas famous? . . . . . . **Opera singing**
5 Which famous actress's real name was Norma Jean Baker? . **Marilyn Monroe**
6 Whose face launched a thousand ships? . . . . . **Helen of Troy**
7 Who said 'I never hated a man long enough to give him back his diamonds'? . . . . **Zsa Zsa Gabor**
8 What was Edith Piaf's nickname? . . . . **The 'little sparrow'**
9 Name the longest reigning British monarch. . . . . . **Queen Victoria**
10 In tennis which woman has won the most titles at Wimbledon? . **Billie Jean King**
11 Which film actress who starred in *High Society* married Prince Rainier of Monaco? . . . . **Grace Kelly**

12	Which novelist created the detective Hercule Poirot? . . .	**Agatha Christie**
13	Who did Edward VIII abdicate to marry?	**Wallis Simpson**
14	In what profession was Margot Fonteyn well known? . . .	**Ballet dancing**
15	What was the name of the famous slender model from London in the 1960s?	**Twiggy**
16	Which authoress wrote about Squirrel Nutkin and Mrs Tiggy-winkle?	**Beatrix Potter**
17	Which famous American child star of *The Little Princess* later became a US ambassador?	**Shirley Temple-Black**
18	Which American social worker, who although both deaf and blind, travelled all over the world giving lectures and campaigning for improvement in the teaching of the physically handicapped? .	**Helen Keller**
19	Which British actress won academy awards for her roles in *Women in Love* and *A Touch of Class*?	**Glenda Jackson**
20	Name the Brontë sisters	**Charlotte, Emily, Anne**

LEVEL C

1	Who was Tutankhamen's mother-in-law?	**Nefertiti**
2	Who was Coco Chanel?	**Dress designer**
3	Who was Amelia Earhart?	**First woman to make a solo flight across the Atlantic**
4	Who was the first female Prime Minister of Israel?	**Golda Meir**
5	Which great woman scientist was awarded two Nobel Prizes in the early years of the twentieth century?	**Marie Curie**
6	Who was Henry VIII's second wife?	**Anne Boleyn**
7	Which woman, dedicated to the relief of the poor, won the 1979 Nobel Peace Prize?	**Mother Teresa**
8	Who, at the age of 43, became the world's first female President and the youngest head of state in Latin America in the 1970s? .	**Marie Estela Isabel Peron**
9	What did Isadora Duncan do to become famous?	**Danced**
10	Which famous poet's wife wrote the novel of horror *Frankenstein: or, The Modern Prometheus*?	**Mary Shelley**

Places of Interest: Europe

LEVEL A

1 In which city would you find the Eiffel Tower? . . . . . **Paris**

2 Where are the crown jewels on show? . . . . . **Tower of London**

3 Where would you go to see the famous leaning tower? . . . **Pisa**

4 Where in Europe would you go to see a bullfight? . . . **Spain**

5 Which Scottish loch is famous for its monster? . . . . **Loch Ness**

6 Which sea washes the southern coasts of Spain, France and Italy? **Mediterranean**

7 In which city would you find the Royal Albert Hall? . . . . **London**

8 Name the two most famous university towns in England . . **Oxford and Cambridge**

9 Which country is known as The Emerald Isle? . . . . **Ireland**

10 People visit the Alps to ski. In which countries are they? . . . **Switzerland, Austria, Italy and France**

LEVEL B

1 Where would you find the Royal Shakespeare Theatre? . . . **Stratford-upon-Avon, England**

2 Which is the smallest independent state in Europe and the world? **The Vatican**

3 The Spanish town of Toledo has long been noted for the manufacture of what? . . . . **High quality steel swords**

4 Stockholm is the capital of which country? . . . . . **Sweden**

5 Name the oldest city in Germany which lies on the left bank of the river Rhine. . . . . **Cologne**

6 In which country are the European Courts of Justice? . . . **Luxembourg**

7 Where would you find The Blarney Stone? . . . . . **County Cork, Ireland**

8 In which city would you find the Brandenburg Gate? . . . **Berlin**

9 In which country would you find the prehistoric monument, Stonehenge? . . . . **England**

10 Which former home of Madame de Pompadour became the official residence of the French President in 1873? . . . . **Elysée Palace**

11	In which country would you find Lake Garda?	**Italy**
12	Which capital city is built on the banks of the river Tiber? . .	**Rome**
13	In which country would you find Lake Geneva?	**Switzerland**
14	If you were sailing on The Broads where would you be? . .	**Norfolk, England**
15	In London it is the underground, in New York it is the subway. What is it in Paris?	**Metro**
16	In which country does the river Danube rise?	**Germany, in the Black Forest**
17	In which country would you be able to visit the Acropolis? .	**Greece**
18	Which country attracts visitors to view its spring bulbs? . .	**Holland (Netherlands)**
19	Which European capital stands on the river Liffey? . . .	**Dublin**
20	What is the main town in the principality of Monaco? . .	**Monte Carlo**

LEVEL C

1	Which feature of the Cathedral of Chartres in France is famous? .	**Its stained glass**
2	Name the deepest lake in Europe.	**Lake Como**
3	What is the name of the artists' quarter in Paris? . . .	**Montmartre**
4	Mozart's birthplace is in which Austrian town? . . .	**Salzburg**
5	On which river does the city of Vienna stand? . . .	**Danube**
6	In which mountain range would you find Mont Blanc? . .	**The Alps**
7	Where was the principal residence of the kings of France? .	**Versailles**
8	The highest active volcano in Europe is situated on an island in the Mediterranean Sea. What is the volcano called? . . .	**Mount Etna**
9	Which French river is famed for the chateaux in its valley? .	**Loire**
10	In which European capital is Wenceslas Square?	**Prague, Czech Republic**

Places of Interest: Rest of World

LEVEL A

1 In which country are the pyramids? . . . . **Egypt**
2 Which famous monument stands in New York harbour? . . . **Statue of Liberty**
3 On which Hawaiian island is Waikiki Beach? . . . . . **Oahu**
4 Where do women wear Kimonos? . . . . **Japan**
5 What was built on the site of the old Waldorf Astoria hotel in New York? . . . . **The Empire State Building**
6 What is the highest mountain in the world? . . . . . **Mount Everest**
7 In which country would you find the Taj Mahal? . . . . **India**
8 Where are the Niagara Falls? . . . . **North America (between Canada and USA)**
9 Which is the longest river in the world? . . . . . . **The Nile**
10 Where would you find the Bronx? . . . . **New York**

LEVEL B

1 Where would you find the Yangtze river? . . . . . . **China**
2 Which country was formerly East Pakistan? . . . . . **Bangladesh**
3 Name the largest Canadian province. . . . . **Quebec**
4 Where is Table Mountain? . . . . **Cape Town, South Africa**
5 In which city is the Blue Mosque? . . . . **Istanbul**
6 Name the bridge that spans San Francisco harbour. . . . **Golden Gate Bridge**
7 On which coast would you find The Great Barrier Reef? . . . **Queensland, Australia**
8 Of which country is Mombasa the chief port? . . . . **Kenya**
9 Where is Cape Horn? . . . . **Southern tip of South America**
10 In which state of the US is the Grand Canyon? . . . . . **Arizona**

11 In which country would you find geisha girls? . . . . . **Japan**

12 From where are American space probes launched? . . . . **Cape Canaveral, Florida**

13 Where is the wailing wall? . . . . **Jerusalem**

14 Near which city is Hollywood? . . . . **Los Angeles**

15 In which country is the port of Alexandria? . . . . . **Egypt**

16 The Rio Grande river forms part of the international boundary
between the US and which country? . . . . **Mexico**

17 Into which sea does the river Nile flow? . . . . . . **Mediterranean**

18 In which country would you find The Great Wall? . . . . **China**

19 Which is the largest mountain range in North America? . . . **The Rockies**

20 In which country would you find Sugar Loaf Mountain? . . . **Brazil**

LEVEL C

1 In which ocean are the Maldive Islands? . . . . . . **Indian Ocean**

2 What is the highest mountain on the continent of Africa? . . **Kilimanjaro**

3 By what name is the largest inland salt water lake in the
world known? . . . . **The Caspian Sea**

4 Which river flows into the Dead Sea? . . . . **River Jordan**

5 Where would you find Ayers Rock? . . . . **Northern Territory, Australia**

6 Which is the lowest area of water in the world? . . . . **Dead Sea**

7 Where would you find the highest waterfall in the world? . . **Venezuela (Angel Falls)**

8 Which canal links the Mediterranean with the Red Sea? . . **The Suez Canal**

9 Which language is spoken in Brazil? . . . . **Portuguese**

10 In which country is Mecca, the holiest city of the
Mohammedean world? . . . . **Saudi Arabia**

Collective Nouns

LEVEL A

Complete the following:

1	A _____ of cows	. Herd
2	A _____ of sheep	. Flock
3	A _____ of pups	. Litter
4	A _____ of wolves	. Pack
5	A _____ of thieves	. Gang
6	An _____ of soldiers	. Army
7	A _____ of grapes . . . . 7 .	. Bunch
8	A _____ of cards	. Deck
9	A _____ of sailors . . . . 9 . A .	. Crew
10	A _____ of people	. Crowd, group

LEVEL B

1	A _____ of fish . . . . 1 .	. Shoal, school
2	A _____ of musicians . . . . 2 . A .	. Band
3	A _____ of geese . . . . 3 .	. Gaggle
4	A _____ of actors . . . . 4 .	. Company, troupe
5	A _____ of chickens . . . . 5 .	. Brood
6	A _____ of wool	. Bale, skein
7	A _____ of birds . . . . 7 .	. Flock
8	A _____ of buffaloes	. Herd
9	A _____ of lions . . . . 9 .	. Pride
10	A _____ of beads	. String

11	A _____ of cotton	Bale
12	A _____ of flowers	Bouquet
13	A _____ of trees	Forest
14	A _____ of hay	Bale
15	A _____ of singers	Choir
16	A _____ of rags	Bundle
17	A _____ of golf clubs	Set
18	A _____ of steps	Flight
19	A _____ of books	Library
20	A _____ of corn	Sheaf

LEVEL C

1	A _____ of mountains	Range
2	A _____ of bees	Swarm
3	A _____ of accidents	Chapter
4	A _____ of ships	Convoy, fleet
5	A _____ of thieves	Den
6	A _____ of diamonds	Cluster
7	A _____ of good luck	Run
8	A _____ of songs	Medley
9	A _____ of partridges	Covey
10	A _____ of shops	Chain

LEVEL A

1 What is the art of taking pictures called? . . . . . **Photography**

2 What is the sport of shooting with a bow called? . . . . **Archery**

3 In which sport would you throw a light spear by hand? . . **Javelin throwing**

4 In which leisure pursuit does a person skim over the surface of the water whilst being towed by a motor boat? . . . . **Water skiing**

5 Ice hockey has its roots in which country? . . . . . **Canada**

6 For what are tarot or taroc cards used? . . . . . . **Fortune telling**

7 What are drivers, spoons, putters and irons? . . . . . **Golf clubs**

8 Which game is played with rackets and a small, fairly soft ball in a closed court? . . . . **Squash**

9 What do you need to play cat's cradle? . . . . . . **A piece of string**

10 What instrument is used in the sport of fencing? . . . . **Foil, epee, sabre**

LEVEL B

1 What are the detachable ends of darts called? . . . . **Flights**

2 In golf, what is a birdie? . . . . **One stroke below par on a hole**

3 In fishing, lines, hooks, floats and weights are known collectively as what? . . . . **Tackle**

4 Which game is played on a lawn with balls, mallets and hoops? . **Croquet**

5 In which game do you knock on the table if you cannot go? . . **Dominoes**

6 How many players are there in an ice hockey team? **6**

7 What is the game where you act out the title of a film, book or play for other players to identify? . . . . **Charades**

8 Sprints, pursuits, road racing, time trials, stage racing and off-road are versions of which sport? . . . . **Cycle racing**

9 In American football, how many points are awarded for a field goal? **3**

10 In what athletic event do the winners move only backwards? . . **Tug-of-war**

11 With what game do you associate triple word scores? . . . **Scrabble®**
12 What do botanists study? . . . . **Plants**
13 In which sport do you play in a small 4-walled room against an opponent and the first to 9 with 2 clear points wins? . . . **Squash**
14 What does an astrologer study? . . . . **Horoscopes**
15 In which sport may asymmetrical bars be used? . . . . **Gymnastics**
16 Who invented a problem cube? . . . . **Rubik**
17 In chess, which piece moves in 'L' shapes? . . . . . **Knight**
18 In which leisure activity is the lotus position assumed? . . . **Yoga**
19 What is the study of the stars and planets called? . . . . **Astronomy**
20 With which hobby do you go on digs? . . . . . . **Archaeology**

LEVEL C

1 When climbing, what would you be doing if you were traversing? **Moving sideways**
2 What is philately? . . . . **Stamp collecting**
3 What does Judo mean? . . . . **The gentle way**
4 Which Chinese game has tiles engraved in suits? . . . . **Mah-jongg**
5 Which popular card game is also known as Vingt-et-un, Blackjack and 21? . . . . **Pontoon**
6 What does a lepidopterist study? . . . . **Butterflies and moths**
7 What is a ski-race down a zig-zag course called? . . . . **Slalom**
8 How many squares are there on a chessboard? **64**
9 How many playing pieces are there in a set of dominoes? . . **28**
10 In golf, what is the traditional name for a number 10 iron? . . **Wedge**

Pets

LEVEL A

1 Which animal is regarded as man's best friend? . . . . **Dog**
2 A dog which does not have a pedigree is known as . . . . **A mongrel, a mutt**
3 What pet did Dick Whittington have in the legend? . . . . **Cat**
4 How do you pick up a mouse? . . . . **Base of the tail with finger and thumb**
5 What is an Alsatian? . . . . **A breed of dog**
6 How many times a day should you feed a goldfish? . . . . **Once**
7 Name the dog in Punch and Judy shows. . . . . . . **Toby**
8 How is the height of a horse measured? . . . . . . **In hands**
9 Which dog resembles the whippet and is used for racing? . . **Greyhound**
10 Siamese, tabby and tortoiseshell are types of what? . . . . **Cat**

LEVEL B

1 Which small animal stores food in its cheek pouches? . . . **Hamster**
2 What colour eyes do Siamese cats have? . . . . . . **Blue**
3 What is a female donkey called? . . . . **A jenny**
4 Which is the smallest breed of dog? . . . . **Chihuahua**
5 How do cats purr? . . . . **Vocal cords vibrate**
6 Why should hamsters be kept in separate cages? . . . . **They fight**
7 Name the tallest breed of dog. . . . . **Irish wolfhound**
8 Which animals might be blue Imperial, New Zealand White or Angora? . . . . **Rabbits**
9 What is a Russian Blue? . . . . **A breed of cat**
10 Why do cats sometimes scratch on furniture? . . . . . **To sharpen their claws**
11 What type of dog do these words describe – Cairn, Jack Russell, Bull and Fox? . . . . **Terrier**

Pets

12 What were husky dogs used for in Iceland and Lapland? . . . **To pull sleds**

13 From what country did the poodle originate? . . . . . **France**

14 What are hens that are kept loose in yards or fields called? . . **Free range**

15 What types of hound are used to hunt hares? . . . . **Beagle and Basset hounds**

16 What is a female mouse called? . . . . **A doe**

17 Name the heaviest breed of domestic dog. . . . . . **St Bernard**

18 What will happen to your goldfish if you leave it in a bowl in a dark room for some weeks? . . . . **It will go pale. If left long enough it will turn white.**

19 Which animal did Joy Adamson write about in her book *Born Free*? . . . . **A lioness (Elsa)**

20 What is the operation to remove the female sex organs of dogs and cats called? . . . . **Spaying**

LEVEL C

1   What are Rainbow fish otherwise known as? . . . . . **Guppies**

2   What is a pregnant cat called? . . . . **A queen**

3   If feline applies to cat and canine applies to dog, what word would apply to a horse? . . . . **Equine**

4   What type of animal is a guinea pig? . . . . . . **Rodent**

5   To which bird family does the canary belong? . . . . **Finch**

6   What is a mule? . . . . **Cross between a horse and a donkey**

7   What kinds of birds are Cushat, Rock and Stock? . . . **Pigeons or doves**

8   What is the name of the small German dog with a long body, drooping ears and short legs? . . . . **Dachshund**

9   What bird makes a wolf whistle sound? . . . . . . **Mynah bird**

10 Snakes have no ears, but as they hear, how do they listen? . . **By constantly flicking their tongues**

LEVEL A

1 Name the tall plant with a round yellow flower which turns to face the sun. . . . . **Sunflower**
2 What is a small spade-like hand tool with a curved blade called? **Trowel**
3 If you find a slimy trail in your garden, which pest has been there? **Slugs or snails**
4 Why do gardeners put nets over their fruit canes? . . . . **To stop the birds picking the fruit**
5 Which fleshy plant with prickles is found in deserts and can be grown in greenhouses? . . . . **Cactus**
6 What colour are forget-me-nots? . . . . **Blue**
7 In which season do crocuses bloom? . . . . **Early spring**
8 What colour are primroses? . . . . **Yellow**
9 Why are flowers perfumed and brightly coloured? . . . **To attract bees and birds**
10 Which tool is used to clear the leaves off the lawn? . . . **Rake**

LEVEL B

1 The cutting out of dead or unwanted parts of a bush or tree is known as what? . . . . **Pruning**
2 What is the popular name for the flowering plant *Impatiens*? . **Busy Lizzy**
3 What sort of soil do rhododendrons like? . . . . . **Acid**
4 What is the most common colour for a peony? . . . . **Pink, red**
5 From which flower does opium come? . . . . . . **Poppy**
6 What is a plant that grows each year without having to be resown called? . . . . **Perennial**
7 Climbers, ramblers and weeping standards are all types of what? **Rose**
8 Why do you put mulch round the bottom of a flower stem? . **Keeps moisture in and provides food for the plant**
9 What does pricking out mean? . . . . **Transplanting from seed boxes to open ground**
10 At what temperature does frost occur? . . . . . . **Below 0°C, 32°F**
11 What colours will hydrangeas growing in acid soil normally be? . **Blue and mauve**

12 Carrots are rich in which vitamin?   .   .   .   .   .   .   **Vitamin C**

13 Tomatoes are grown widely throughout the world but where do
    they originally come from?   .   .   .   .   **Latin America**

14 What is an aphid?   .   .   .   .   **A small insect that is
    destructive to plants**

15 What is chlorophyll?   .   .   .   .   **The substance which
    gives plants their green
    colour**

16 King Edward, Epicu, Majestic, Red King are all types of what?   .   **Potato**

17 What is the name of the art of artificially dwarfing trees?   .   .   **Bonsai**

18 What disease attacks potatoes and caused the Irish potato famine
    of 1846?   .   .   .   .   **Potato blight**

19 What are Fennel, Basil and Marjoram?   .   .   .   .   .   .   **Herbs**

20 Where would you grow the following plants – Clematis,   **Up a wall or fence (all
    Jasmine and Wistaria?   .   .   .   .   climbers)**

LEVEL C

1   By what name is the Lima or Madagascar bean often known?   .   **Butter bean**

2   What is a hybrid?   .   .   .   .   **Offspring of two different
    species or varieties**

3   What is a biennial?   .   .   .   .   **A plant that completes
    its life cycle in two
    growing seasons**

4   What is the cup or trumpet of a daffodil or narcissus called?   .   **Corona**

5   What is a tine?   .   .   .   .   **One of the prongs of a
    garden fork or rake**

6   Which vegetable is hollowed out and used as a lantern at
    Halloween?   .   .   .   .   **Pumpkin**

7   What type of garden peas are most used for canning and freezing?   **Marrowfat**

8   What is the art of training and cutting plants into ornamental
    shapes called?   .   .   .   .   **Topiary**

9   What is the more common name for the *digitalis purpurea*?   .   .   **Foxglove**

10 What is the name of the pollen-producing part of a flower?   .   .   **Anther**

Entertainers

LEVEL A

1 Complete the following: The Keystone . . . . **Cops** ✓
2 Who is 007? . . . . **James Bond** ✓
3 Complete the following: Abbot and . . . . **Costello** ✓
4 Who are Kermit, Fozzie and Miss Piggy? . . . . . **Muppets** ✓
5 Who did Bob Hope partner in many comedy films? . . . **Bing Crosby** ✓
6 What sort of person did Charlie Chaplin generally depict in his films? . . . . **A tramp** ✓
7 What type of dog was Lassie? . . . . **Collie** ✓
8 Who played Dorothy in the film *The Wizard of Oz*? . . . **Judy Garland** ✓
9 Where did the Beatles come from? . . . . . . **Liverpool** ✓
10 Who is Mickey Mouse's girlfriend? . . . . . . **Minnie** ✓

LEVEL B

1 What was the name of Clark Gable's last film? . . . . . *The Misfits*
2 What instrument did Benny Goodman play? . . . . . . **Clarinet**
3 Who was Marilyn Monroe's last husband? . . . . . . **Arthur Miller**
4 In which film do Jack Lemmon and Tony Curtis dress in drag? . *Some Like It Hot*
5 Who says 'Another fine mess you got me into'? . . . . . **Oliver Hardy to Stan Laurel**
6 Which two great actors starred in the film *Butch Cassidy and the Sundance Kid*? . . . . **Robert Redford and Paul Newman**
7 Who sang about the *Green Green Grass of Home*? . . . . **Tom Jones** ✓
8 Which female singer is a *Big Spender*? . . . . . . **Shirley Bassey** ✓
9 Who wrote the music for *Evita*, *Cats* and *Phantom of the Opera*? **Andrew Lloyd-Webber**
10 What was Princess Grace of Monaco's name before she married? **Grace Kelly** ✓
11 Name David Attenborough's actor and director brother. . . . **Richard**

12 Which actress wanted to wash that man right out of her hair
in the film *South Pacific*? . . . . **Mitzi Gaynor**

13 Which popular American conductor went missing presumed dead
after a plane crash when travelling from France to England? . . **Glen Miller**

14 Who played J R Ewing in the TV series *Dallas*? . . . . **Larry Hagman**

15 Which instrument do you associate with Louis Armstrong? . . **Trumpet**

16 Who did Mia Farrow marry in 1966? . . . . **Frank Sinatra**

17 Who had a big hit in the 1930s with *A Tisket, a Tasket*? . . . **Ella Fitzgerald**

18 Which famous actress was married to Humphrey Bogart? . . **Lauren Bacall**

19 Which famous man directed the film *The Birds*? . . . . . **Alfred Hitchcock**

20 Which singer/dancer/actor danced in the rain in the film *Singin'
In The Rain*? . . . . **Gene Kelly**

LEVEL C

1 Who spent much of her screen career in the water? . . . . **Esther Williams**

2 Gene Krupa became widely acclaimed as the greatest jazz
musician on what instrument? . . . . **Drums**

3 To whom was Mike Todd married when he was killed in a plane
crash in 1958? . . . . **Elizabeth Taylor**

4 Who is Warren Beatty's actress sister? . . . . . . **Shirley Maclaine**

5 Who sang *Wandrin' Star* in the film *Paint Your Wagon*? . . **Lee Marvin**

6 Where was Bob Hope born? . . . . **London (Eltham)**

7 In the film *Grand Hotel* which actress said 'I want to be alone'? . **Greta Garbo**

8 The most decorated American soldier in the Second World War
became a famous film star. Who was he? . . . . . . **Audie Murphy**

9 Who plays Lieutenant Columbo in the TV series *Columbo*? . **Peter Falk**

10 He starred in *Annie Get Your Gun*, *Seven Brides for Seven Brothers*
and *Showboat*. Who is he? . . . . **Howard Keel**

Similes

LEVEL A

1 As blind as a . . . . bat
2 As busy as a . . . . bee or ant
3 As good as . . . . As gold
4 As green as . . . . grass
5 As light as a . . . . feather
6 As fresh as a . . . . daisy
7 As fat as a . . . . pig
8 As black as . . . . coal or sin
9 As dead as a . . . . doornail
10 As sober as a . . . . judge

LEVEL B

1 As dry as a . . . . bone or dust
2 As heavy as . . . . lead
3 As playful as a . . . . kitten
4 As graceful as a . . . . swan
5 As right as . . . . rain
6 As pretty as a . . . . picture
7 As obstinate as a . . . . mule
8 As thin as a . . . . rake
9 As true as . . . . gospel
10 As thick as . . . . thieves

Similes

11	As hard as	**nails**
12	As keen as	**mustard**
13	As slippery as an	**eel**
14	As hungry as a	**wolf**
15	As strong as an	**ox or horse**
16	As sound as a	**bell**
17	As wise as an	**owl**
18	As white as a	**sheet or snow**
19	As clean as a	**whistle**
20	As sour as	**vinegar or grapes**

LEVEL C

1	As easy as	**ABC or winking**
2	As sturdy as an	**oak**
3	As fit as a	**fiddle**
4	As bold as	**brass**
5	As large as	**life**
6	As deep as the	**ocean**
7	As cheap as	**dirt**
8	As smooth as	**clockwork**
9	As old as	**Methuselah or the hills**
10	As flat as a	**pancake**

LEVEL A

1 Which is the hardest stone? . . . . **Diamond**
2 How can you tell the age of a tree? . . . . **By the number of rings in the trunk**
3 What instrument is used to study minute particles at close quarters? . . . . **Microscope**
4 What kind of acid is normally used in a car battery? . . . **Sulphuric Acid**
5 What happens to a bee once it has stung something or someone? **It dies**
6 What is H_2O? . . . . **Water**
7 What is the common name for sodium chloride? . . . . **Salt**
8 When might you see a rainbow? . . . . **When it is raining and the sun is shining**
9 What element provided power for mills apart from wind? . . **Water**
10 What is a deciduous tree? . . . . **One that sheds its leaves annually**

LEVEL B

1 What is the study of weather called? . . . . **Meteorology**
2 Beer is brewed: how is whisky produced? . . . . . **Distilled**
3 Which planet appears to be red? . . . . **Mars**
4 What is the process by which green plants manufacture food from inorganic materials with the help of light? . . . . . **Photosynthesis**
5 Between the stages of caterpillar and butterfly, what state is the insect in? . . . . **Pupa, chrysalis**
6 What is a conch? . . . . **A shell**
7 What does carnivorous mean? . . . . **Flesh eating**
8 What is the name of the single-celled animal? . . . . . **Amoeba**
9 On what are earthquakes measured? . . . . . **The Richter Scale**
10 Which metal is liquid at ordinary temperature? . . . . **Mercury**

11	What colour would litmus paper turn if dipped in acid? . . .	**Red**
12	What is arable land?	**Land which is ploughed and sown with crops**
13	How many carats has pure gold?	**24**
14	By what name is solid carbon dioxide known?	**Dry ice**
15	At what temperature in Fahrenheit does water freeze? . . .	**32°F**
16	What are Leopard, Emperor and Speckled Yellow?	**Breeds of butterfly**
17	What is cumulus?	**Cloud**
18	Which metal, when in ribbon or powder form, burns with a brilliant white light?	**Magnesium**
19	What way does the needle on a compass point?	**North**
20	Which fruit has its seeds on the outside?	**Strawberry**

LEVEL C

1	What is the chemical process which hardens rubber? . . .	**Vulcanization**
2	What is ichthyology?	**The study of fishes**
3	What are the three constituents of an atom?	**Proton, electron and neutron**
4	How hard must the wind blow to be called a hurricane? . .	**More than 75 mph**
5	What does the chemical symbol K represent?	**Potassium**
6	What is royal jelly?	**A rich substance created by the worker bees for the queen**
7	What is the name for the group of plants which obtain their nitrogen from animal tissue?	**Carnivorous or insectivorous**
8	What colour is bromide?	**Brown**
9	Canvas, rope and sailcloth are made from which plant? . . .	**Hemp**
10	Name the toxic substance that comes from the exhaust of vehicles.	**Carbon monoxide**

Myths, Tales & Legends

LEVEL A

1. Who slayed a dragon and became a saint? . . . . . **(St) George**
2. Where did Robin Hood and his merry men live? . . . . **Sherwood Forest**
3. Which king pulled a sword out of a stone? . . . . **Arthur**
4. Who climbed a beanstalk? . . . . **Jack**
5. On which night of the year are witches said to take to their brooms? . . . . **Hallowe'en, 31 October**
6. What did Cinderella leave behind when she fled from the ball? **A glass slipper**
7. Who killed Cock Robin? . . . . **Sparrow**
8. Who was Hansel's partner in the fairy tale? . . . . **Gretel**
9. Whatever he touched turned into gold: who was he? . . **King Midas**
10. Who does the legend say lived in a castle in Transylvania? . **Count Dracula**

LEVEL B

1. Who had snakes for hair? . . . . **Medusa**
2. Who shot an apple off his son's head? . . . . . **William Tell**
3. Which planet was named after the goddess of love? . . . **Venus**
4. Name the Roman equivalent of the love god Eros? . . . **Cupid**
5. Who was condemned to carry the world on his shoulders for making war on the Gods? . . . . **Atlas**
6. Who did Diana fall in love with and Apollo trick her into shooting, thus changing him into a custer of stars? . . . . . **Orion**
7. In which part of the world is the Abominable Snowman said to roam? . . . . **Himalayas**
8. What was the occupation of Snow White's seven dwarfs? . **Diamond miners**
9. Which Roman slave drew a thorn out of a lion's paw and was saved when it recognised him in the arena? . . . . . **Androcles**
10. What was released from Pandora's box? . . . . . **Evil spirits**
11. Name Sundance's partner in crime? . . . . . . **Butch Cassidy**
12. Name Jason's compatriots who sought the Golden Fleece. . **Argonauts**

13 Who flew too near the sun and drowned when the wax in his wings melted? . . . . **Icarus**

14 Which legendary monster was kept in a labyrinth? . . . . **Minotaur**

15 How did Cleopatra die? . . . . **Bitten by an asp**

16 Which Indian brave asked Nokomis, his grandmother, questions about life? . . . . **Hiawatha**

17 Who had a magic hammer which returned to his hand when he threw it at an enemy? . . . . **Thor**

18 Who was King Arthur's wife? . . . . **Guinevere**

19 Who was the Danish author of many fairy tales including *The Little Mermaid*? . . . . **Anderson**

20 In which of Shakespeare's plays are there three witches? . . **Macbeth**

LEVEL C

1 Who gave Theseus the thread which enabled him to find his way out of the labyrinth? . . . . **Ariadne**

2 Name the monster that the Danish warrior Beowulf killed. . . **Grendel**

3 What was the animal which guarded the gates to Hades called? **Cerberus**

4 Which epic poet wrote the *Iliad* and the *Odyssey*? . . . . **Homer**

5 Name the most famous Greek hero of the Trojan war? . . . **Achilles**

6 Which legendary character fished in the sea for islands? . . **Maui**

7 In folklore, what name is given to the sea-creature which has the body of a woman and the tail of a fish? . . . . . . **Mermaid**

8 What was William Bonney better known as? . . . . . **Billy the Kid**

9 Who fell in love with his own reflection, took his own life and was turned into a flower? . . . . **Narcissus**

10 How did the custom of celebrating Christmas on 25 December begin? . . . . **Originally Christ's birth was celebrated on 6 January. In the 4th century the Church moved it to replace the pagan mid-winter festival**

Capital Cities

LEVEL A

1	United Kingdom	**London**
2	France	**Paris**
3	Greece	**Athens**
4	Holland (Netherlands)	**Amsterdam**
5	Israel	**Jerusalem**
6	Belgium	**Brussels**
7	Japan	**Tokyo**
8	Russian Federation	**Moscow**
9	Italy	**Rome**
10	India	**New Delhi**
11	Irish Republic	**Dublin**
12	USA	**Washington DC**
13	Poland	**Warsaw**
14	Iran	**Tehran**
15	Portugal	**Lisbon**

LEVEL B

1	New Zealand	**Wellington**
2	Argentina	**Buenos Aires**
3	Hungary	**Budapest**
4	Malaysia	**Kuala Lumpur**
5	Turkey	**Ankara**
6	Sweden	**Stockholm**
7	Egypt	**Cairo**
8	Norway	**Oslo**
9	Peru	**Lima**
10	Czech Republic	**Prague**
11	Ghana	**Accra**
12	Thailand	**Bangkok**
13	Kenya	**Nairobi**
14	Jamaica	**Kingston**

15	Tunisia	. . . .	**Tunis**
16	Denmark	. . . .	**Copenhagen**
17	Cuba	. . . .	**Havana**
18	Bulgaria	. . . .	**Sofia**
19	China	. . . .	**Beijing (Peking)**
20	Nigeria	. . . .	**Lagos**
21	Yugoslavia	. . . .	**Belgrade**
22	Lebanon	. . . .	**Beirut**
23	Switzerland	. . . .	**Berne**
24	Austria	. . . .	**Vienna**
25	Finland	. . . .	**Helsinki**
26	Iraq	. . . .	**Baghdad**
27	Australia	. . . .	**Canberra**
28	Canada	. . . .	**Ottawa**
29	Germany	. . . .	**Berlin**
30	Romania	. . . .	**Bucharest**

LEVEL C

1	Liechtenstein	. . . .	**Vaduz**
2	Bahamas	. . . .	**Nassau**
3	Uruguay	. . . .	**Montevideo**
4	Botswana	. . . .	**Gaborone**
5	Qatar	. . . .	**Doha**
6	Albania	. . . .	**Tirana**
7	Bahrain	. . . .	**Manama**
8	Honduras	. . . .	**Tegucigalpa**
9	Western Samoa	. . . .	**Apia**
10	Sierra Leone	. . . .	**Freetown**
11	Venezuela	. . . .	**Caracas**
12	Malawi	. . . .	**Lilongwe**
13	Paraguay	. . . .	**Asuncion**
14	Saudi Arabia	. . . .	**Riyadh**
15	Philippines	. . . .	**Manila**

Animals

LEVEL A

1	Which is the tallest of all living mammals?	**Giraffe**
2	One animal is regarded as king among beasts: name it.	**Lion**
3	Puppy is to dog as tadpole is to	**Frog**
4	How many legs has a spider?	**8**
5	Name the largest living animal.	**Whale**
6	What is a flounder?	**Fish**
7	Where is a scorpion's sting?	**In its tail**
8	Which animal eats nothing but bamboo shoots?	**Panda**
9	How does a hedgehog protect itself?	**With its spines – curls up in a ball**
10	From which country does the kangaroo come?	**Australia**

LEVEL B

1	Some animals sleep through the winter: what is this known as?	**Hibernation**
2	In which country would you find koala bears?	**Australia**
3	What is the name given to mammals who carry their young in an external pouch?	**Marsupial**
4	Which is the fastest animal on earth?	**Cheetah**
5	Name the only mammal that can truly fly?	**Bat**
6	Which mythical animal had the body of a horse and a long twisted horn in the middle of its forehead?	**Unicorn**
7	Name the world's largest snake.	**Anaconda**
8	What is a gecko?	**A species of lizard**
9	What type of creature is a sidewinder?	**A desert rattlesnake**
10	To what group of animals do frogs belong?	**Amphibians**
11	How has nature helped the reindeer to travel over snow?	**Wide hooves**
12	Name the first animal to be found in the dictionary.	**Aardvark**

13 Name the largest member of the deer family.   **Elk or moose**

14 Which animal is known as the ship of the desert?   **The camel**

15 Which animal is used as a beast of burden in some Latin American countries apart from horses and donkeys?   **Llama**

16 What is the name given to the Arabian camel with one hump?   **Dromedary**

17 Give another name for the coyote   **Prairie wolf**

18 What is a triceratops?   **A dinosaur**

19 By what name is the parasitic insect *pulex irritans* more commonly known?   **The human flea**

20 Where do tigers come from?   **India**

LEVEL C

1 How many legs has a lobster?   **10**

2 Are bats blind?   **No**

3 What do the snake and stick symbols of the medicine profession signify?   **The snake represents wisdom and the stick is the staff of Aesculapius, the ancient god of medicine**

4 What is so unusual about the chameleon?   **It can change its colour**

5 What is a caiman?   **A species of crocodile found in Latin America**

6 What kind of animal is a basilisk?   **Lizard**

7 What is a charolais?   **A French breed of cow**

8 Name the largest living amphibian?   **Giant salamander**

9 Which species of cat has tufted ears and cheek ruffs which distinguish it from other cats?   **Lynx**

10 How do millipedes protect themselves?   **By giving out a smell**

Birds

LEVEL A

1   What did 'my true love' send me on the first day of Christmas?   . **A partridge in a pear tree**
2   Which birds are used to carry messages?   . . . . . **Pigeons**
3   'One for sorrow, two for joy, three for a girl, four for a boy.' With which bird is this rhyme associated?   . . . . . **Magpie**
4   Which bird's call is associated with the coming of spring in Britain?   . . . . **Cuckoo**
5   Some birds come and go with the seasons of the year. What is this behaviour known as?   . . . . **Migration**
6   Which bird is usually illustrated on Christmas cards?   . . . **Robin**
7   Which bird is associated with the birth of children?   . . . . **Stork**
8   Which duck is associated with quilts?   . . . . . . **Eider**
9   What is a male duck called?   . . . . **Drake**
10 Which bird is traditionally known as the farmyard alarm clock?   . **Rooster**

LEVEL B

1   Which bird fishes in shallow water using the vast pouch under its bill as a drag net?   . . . . **Pelican**
2   Which bird did Noah first release from the ark?   . . . . **Raven**
3   What is the name of the laughing bird of Australia?   . . . **Kookaburra**
4   Which bird is associated with wisdom?   . . . . . . **Owl**
5   Name the largest bird in the world.   . . . . . . **Ostrich**
6   What is the name given to a large showy bird's feather?   . . . **Plume**
7   One bird has the traditional status of being king amongst birds: name it.   . . . . **Golden eagle**
8   Which flightless bird lives only in the southern polar region?   . **Penguin**
9   An eagle's nest is called an   . . . . **Eyrie**
10 What is the flightless bird from New Zealand called?   . . . . **Kiwi**
11 What type of bird is a mallard?   . . . . **Duck**

12 How can you tell the difference between a male blackbird and a female? . . . . **The female blackbird is brown**

13 Which birds is the Tower of London famous for? . . . . **Ravens**

14 Which bird in flight has the largest wing span? . . . . **Albatross**

15 In the 17th century a breed of bird on Mauritius became extinct. Name it. . . . . **Dodo**

16 Why do birds sing? . . . . **It is how they communicate with each other**

17 In which country would you find emus? . . . . . . **Australia**

18 Which bird climbs trees and chisels through the wood to find insects? . . . . **Woodpecker**

19 Which bird can hibernate? . . . . **None**

20 From which country did the turkey originate? . . . . . **North America**

LEVEL C

1 How did the mockingbird get its name? . . . . **It mimics other birds**

2 What is the name of the large vulture of the Andes which attacks young animals? . . . . **Condor**

3 Which bird cremated itself every 500 years and rose rejuvenated from its own ashes? . . . . **Phoenix**

4 What are *sturnus vulgaris* commonly known as? . . . . . **Starlings**

5 By what name is the blue peafowl commonly known? . . . **Peacock**

6 What are birds and animals called that sleep during the day and hunt for their food at night? . . . . **Nocturnal**

7 Which bird of prey is the most successful and efficient at fishing? **Osprey**

8 From where do humming birds derive their name? . . . . **The sound of their wings rapidly beating**

9 Which is the only bird that can fly backwards and hover? . . **The humming bird**

10 Which birds has its nostrils at the end of its beak? . . . . **The kiwi**

Proverbs & Sayings

LEVEL A

1	A penny for your	thoughts
2	Too many cooks spoil the	broth
3	Two's company three's a	crowd
4	There's no smoke without	fire
5	First come first	served
6	Easy come easy	go
7	The early bird catches the	worm
8	A rolling stone gathers	no moss
9	Absence makes the heart	grow fonder
10	Early to bed, early to rise, makes a man healthy, wealthy and	wise
11	It never rains but it	pours
12	Honesty is the best	policy
13	It's no use crying over spilt	milk
14	All's well that ends	well
15	Let sleeping dogs	lie

LEVEL B

1	Children should be seen	but not heard
2	A stitch in time	saves nine
3	Fools rush in	where angels fear to tread
4	People who live in glass houses	should not throw stones
5	Empty vessels	make most noise
6	A bird in the hand	is worth two in the bush
7	Red sky at night, shepherd's delight	Red sky in the morning, shepherd's warning
8	He who laughs last	laughs longest
9	Jack of all trades	master of none
10	More haste	less speed
11	All that glitters	is not gold
12	An apple a day	keeps the doctor away
13	In for a penny	in for a pound
14	Still waters	run deep

Proverbs & Sayings

15	Where there is life	there is hope
16	A poor workman	always blames his tools
17	Birds of a feather	flock together
18	Every cloud	has a silver lining
19	Mighty oaks	from little acorns grow
20	You can't teach an old dog	new tricks
21	Curiosity	killed the cat
22	You can't put new wine	in old bottles
23	You can lead a horse to water	but you can't make it drink
24	Marry in haste	repent at leisure
25	The course of true love	never did run smooth
26	United we stand	divided we fall
27	A friend in need	is a friend indeed
28	Penny wise	pound foolish
29	Enough is as good	as a feast
30	While the cat's away	the mice will play

LEVEL C

1	Time	and tide wait for no man
2	Pride	comes before a fall
3	Misery acquaints a man with	strange bedfellows
4	To err	is human, to forgive divine
5	One swallow	does not make a summer
6	Every dog	has his day
7	Practice makes	perfect
8	Actions speak louder	than words
9	You can't paint	black white
10	You can't make a silk	purse out of a sow's ear
11	A change	is as good as a rest
12	Necessity	is the mother of invention
13	Robbing	Peter to pay Paul
14	Casting pearls	before swine
15	Fortune	knocks once at every man's door

LEVEL A

1 On what does an artist rest the canvas while painting?   .   .   . **An easel**
2 What is a mural?   .   .   .   . **Any form of wall painting or ceiling decoration**

3 If you mix yellow and blue paint together what happens?   . **It turns green**
4 What happens to brushes if they are left in enamel paint?   . **They go hard and cannot be used**

5 With what did the first artists draw?   .   .   .   .   .   . **Rocks**
6 What colour is buff?   .   .   .   . **Fawn**
7 Which city is regarded as the world centre for fashion?   .   . **Paris**
8 In what type of building are pictures displayed to the public?   . **Art gallery**
9 Which film cartoonist created Mickey Mouse?   .   .   .   . **Walt Disney**
10 Which two colours mixed together make orange?   .   .   . **Yellow and red**

LEVEL B

1 Who painted *The Last Supper*?   .   .   .   . **Leonardo da Vinci**
2 To what school of painting did the artists Renoir, Degas and Monet belong?   .   .   .   . **The Impressionists**
3 Which nationality was Rembrandt?   .   .   .   .   .   . **Dutch**
4 Name the famous Spanish surrealist painter   .   .   .   .   . **Salvador Dali**
5 Which French painter visited Polynesia and painted *The Tahitian Woman*?   .   .   .   . **Paul Gauguin**
6 Which Dutch painter cut off his ear?   .   .   .   .   .   . **Vincent van Gogh**
7 Which Spanish artist evolved a new style called cubism?   .   . **Pablo Picasso**
8 What is a collage?   .   .   .   . **Different fabric etc, glued to a back cloth, to make a picture**

9 What colour is puce?   .   .   .   . **Brownish purple**
10 What is the Japanese art-form of paper folding called?   .   .   . **Origami**
11 In what type of art would you use acid, wax and needles?   .   . **Etching**

12	What colours make a scene appear to recede in a picture?	**Blues and violets**
13	How do you mix the colour brown?	**Red, yellow and black or blue**
14	What type of painting do the French refer to as *nature morte* and the Spanish *bodegan*?	**Still life**
15	Who did a series of paintings of young men and light reflecting in water?	**David Hockney**
16	Where is the *Mona Lisa* hung?	**Louvre art gallery, Paris**
17	What is a mosaic?	**A pattern or picture made with small pieces of glass or stone of different colours**
18	What is an icon?	**Religious portrait**
19	Who painted *The Blue Boy*?	**Thomas Gainsborough**
20	Which great French sculptor created *The Kiss* and *The Thinker*?	**Rodin**

LEVEL C

1	Some sculptors use bronze. What is this an alloy of?	**Copper and tin**
2	Which English artist painted *The Rake's Progress*?	**William Hogarth**
3	What sort of works of art did El Greco paint?	**Religious**
4	Who was the illustrator of Lewis Carroll's book, *Alice in Wonderland*?	**Sir John Tenniel**
5	Who was Jacob Epstein?	**A sculptor**
6	What is gouache?	**Non-transparent water colour paint that provides easy way of obtaining oil painting effect**
7	What is a fresco?	**Painting made on wet plaster**
8	Who made a famous statue of David?	**Michelangelo**
9	Who painted *The Laughing Cavalier*?	**Frans Hals**
10	Which French painter was dwarfed because of an accident to his legs?	**Toulouse-Lautrec**

Spelling

LEVEL A

1. Ache
2. Friend
3. Rule
4. Under
5. Lamb
6. Event
7. Cycle
8. Apron
9. Half
10. Very
11. Town
12. Heat
13. Tax
14. Farm
15. Mother
16. Crab
17. Book
18. Milk
19. Jazz
20. Apple
21. High
22. News
23. Flood
24. Egg
25. Star
26. Lion
27. Sport
28. Church
29. Pass
30. People
31. Nose
32. Truck
33. House
34. Decide
35. Blank
36. Herb
37. Butter
38. Five
39. Small
40. River

LEVEL B

1. Solemn
2. Convenient
3. Friction
4. Excellent
5. Pigeon
6. Symptom
7. Adjourn
8. Resurrection
9. Receive
10. Profession
11. Infamous
12. Pharmacy
13. Exhibition
14. Phoenix
15. Obnoxious
16. Nostalgia
17. Middleweight
18. Patience
19. Luggage
20. Juggernaut
21. Irritate
22. Aggressive
23. Lattice
24. Immunize
25. Harlequin
26. Grotesque
27. Freight
28. Drought
29. Possession
30. Curriculum
31. Nautical
32. Grievous
33. Vague
34. Platypus
35. Nicaragua
36. Squirrel
37. Conquer
38. Caterpillar
39. Moustache

40 Crystals	55 Vaccine	70 Cryptic
41 Instruments	56 Atmosphere	71 Quadraphonic
42 Beethoven	57 Carbohydrate	72 Bailiff
43 Necessary	58 Architecture	73 Criticism
44 Procession	59 Buddha	74 Apostrophe
45 Thatched	60 Chimpanzee	75 Sapphire
46 Cough	61 Cosmonaut	76 Antenna
47 Recipe	62 Accommodation	77 Crustacean
48 Audience	63 Syllabus	78 Obituary
49 Oxygen	64 Business	79 Guarantee
50 Cuckoo	65 Penicillin	80 Hawaii
51 Cipher	66 Marquee	
52 Millipede	67 Environment	
53 Chameleon	68 Exhaust	
54 Porpoise	69 Decipher	

LEVEL C

1 Panache	15 Hypochondria	29 Freesia
2 Czechoslovakia	16 Dachshund	30 Fujiyama
3 Miscellaneous	17 Bolognaise	31 Rhapsody
4 Ostracize	18 Moccasin	32 Fallacy
5 Luminescent	19 Reorientate	33 Onomatopoeia
6 Whimsical	20 Loofah	34 Kilohertz
7 Jodhpurs	21 Hieroglyphics	35 Sulphuric
8 Guillotine	22 Euphonium	36 Dyslexia
9 Garrulous	23 Dissertation	37 Lieutenant
10 Jeopardize	24 Bourgeois	38 Ambidextrous
11 Therapeutic	25 Rhetoric	39 Liaison
12 Masseur	26 Discrepancy	40 Deutschmark
13 Mannequin	27 Pseudonym	
14 Afghanistan	28 Susceptible	

Medical Matters

LEVEL A

1   Name the instrument used by doctors to listen to the lungs and heart. . . . . **Stethoscope**

2   If this is grumbling it may need to be taken out. What is it? . . **Appendix**

3   What is the instrument for taking a person's temperature? . . **Thermometer**

4   What are Siamese Twins? . . . . **Twin babies which are born joined together**

5   Some people who need to wear glasses wear tiny pieces of plastic directly on their eyes. What are these called? . . . **Contact lenses**

6   If you are allergic to the pollens of certain plants, what are you said to suffer from? . . . . **Hay fever**

7   When a person volunteers to give blood what are they called? . **Donor**

8   What is a migraine? . . . . **A severe type of headache**

9   If someone is obese, what is wrong with them? . . . . **Overweight**

10 Where is the muscle called the biceps? . . . . . . **In the upper arm**

LEVEL B

1   If you suffer from myopia what is the matter? . . . . . **You are short-sighted**

2   Where is the jugular vein? . . . . **In the neck**

3   Approximately how many times do you breathe in a minute? . **16**

4   Platelets are found in the blood: what are their main purpose? . **Cause clotting**

5   What is the name of the alternative medicine that involves the insertion of small needles into parts of the human body? . . **Acupuncture**

6   What is the name of the surgical delivery of a baby when natural childbirth is impossible? . . . . **Caesarean**

7   What is the definition of a squint? . . . . **Both eyes do not point in the same direction**

8   What are fallen arches also called? . . . . **Flat feet**

9   What is vertigo? . . . . **Dizziness**

10 What is the name of the band of tissue that connects a muscle to a bone? . . . . **Tendon**

11   Which deadly disease is passed on by an animal bite?   .   .   .   **Rabies**

12   What is the removal of a small piece of tissue for examination under a microscope called?   .   .   .   .   **Biopsy**

13   What is the common name for the patella?   .   .   .   .   .   **Knee cap**

14   What is the name of the lower bony end of the spinal column?   .   **Coccyx**

15   Scurvy is related to a deficiency of which vitamin?   .   .   .   .   **C**

16   What are the growths of tissue at the back of the throat which are often removed at the same time as the tonsils?   .   .   .   .   .   **Adenoids**

17   What is the main sympton in laryngitis?   .   .   .   .   .   .   **Loss of voice**

18   What is alopecia?   .   .   .   .   **Loss of hair**

19   What is the name of the type of spectacles which have lenses made up of two parts?   .   .   .   .   **Bifocals**

20   What part of the body is affected in pleurisy?   .   .   .   .   .   **Lungs**

LEVEL C

1   What are the four main blood groups?   .   .   .   .   .   .   **A, B, AB and O**

2   What is somnambulism?   .   .   .   .   **Sleep walking**

3   Disorder in what part of the body causes jaundice?   .   .   .   .   **Liver**

4   What type of arthritis commonly affects the big toe?   .   .   .   .   **Gout**

5   Nephritis is infection in which part of the body?   .   .   .   .   .   **Kidneys**

6   Carpal tunnel syndrome causes pain in which part of the body?   .   **Wrist**

7   What is your sternum?   .   .   .   .   **Breast bone**

8   What is Potts Fracture?   .   .   .   .   **Broken ankle**

9   An epidemic disease that spreads to many countries is called what?   .   .   .   .   **Pandemic**

10   What is the common name for rubella?   .   .   .   .   .   .   **German measles**

Male/Female Genders & Their Young

1 What is a male cow called? . . . . **Bull**
2 What is a male hen called? . . . . **Cock**
3 What is a young sheep called? . . . . **Lamb**
4 What is a young horse called? . . . . **Foal**
5 What is a young cat called? . . . . **Kitten**
6 What is a young dog called? . . . . **Puppy**
7 What is a female lion called? . . . . **Lioness**
8 What is a young goat called? . . . . **Kid**
9 What is a female dog called? . . . . **Bitch**
10 What is a female actor called? . . . . **Actress**

LEVEL B

1 What is a female fox called? . . . . **Vixen**
2 What is a female sheep called? . . . . **Ewe**
3 What is a male horse called? . . . . **Stallion**
4 What is a male rabbit called? . . . . **Buck**
5 What is a male witch called? . . . . **Wizard**
6 What is a young whale called? . . . . **Calf**
7 What is a female peafowl called? . . . . **Peahen**
8 What is a young stag called? . . . . **Fawn**
9 What is a male sheep called? . . . . **Ram**
10 What is a young goose called? . . . . **Gosling**

11	What is a young tiger called?	Cub
12	What is a male pig called?	Boar
13	What is the male equivalent of a niece?	Nephew
14	What is the female equivalent of a duke?	Duchess
15	What is a female goat called?	Nanny
16	What is a young frog called?	Tadpole
17	What is a young eel called?	Elver
18	What is the female equivalent of a bachelor?	Spinster
19	What is a female deer called?	Doe
20	What is a young elephant called?	Calf

LEVEL C

1	What is a female ferret called?	Gill
2	What is a female badger called?	Sow
3	What is a young hare called?	Leveret
4	What is a male swan called?	Cob
5	What is a young seal called?	Pup
6	What is a young trout called?	Fry
7	What is a female sultan called?	Sultana
8	What is a young kangaroo called?	Joey
9	What is a young wasp called?	Grub
10	What is a male heifer called?	Steer

Bible

LEVEL A

1 Who had a coat of many colours? . . . . **Joseph**
2 What gifts did the three kings bring to Jesus? . . . . **Gold, frankincense, myrrh**
3 Who according to the Bible killed Goliath? . . . . . **David**
4 What hero was betrayed by Delilah? . . . . **Samson**
5 Who were Jesus' parents? . . . . **Mary and Joseph**
6 Who turned into a pillar of salt? . . . . **Lot's wife**
7 How many commandments was Moses given? **10**
8 What was the name of the disciple who betrayed Jesus? . . **Judas Iscariot**
9 With what did Jesus feed the five thousand? . . . . . **5 loaves and 2 fishes**
10 What did the dove bring back in its beak to the ark? . . . **An olive leaf**

LEVEL B

1 Who asked 'Am I my brother's keeper?' . . . . . . **Cain**
2 The Queen of which country visited Solomon? . . . . **Sheba**
3 Where did Moses receive the Ten Commandments? . . . **Mount Sinai**
4 What is the shortest verse in the Bible? . . . . . . **Jesus wept**
5 Who had a dream about a ladder going up to heaven? . . **Jacob**
6 Where did Noah's ark come to rest after the flood? . . . **Ararat**
7 How many days did Jesus spend in the wilderness without food or water? . . . . **40 days and 40 nights**
8 Name the first book of the Bible. . . . . **Genesis**
9 One disciple was described by Jesus as 'the rock'. Name him. . **Peter**
10 After his conversion to Christianity which name did Saul assume? **Paul**
11 Where did the disciples go fishing? . . . . **Sea of Galilee**
12 Who asked for John the Baptist's head? . . . . . . **Salome**

13	How many tribes of Israel were there?	**12**
14	What miracle did Jesus perform at the wedding in Cana?	**Turned water into wine**
15	Complete the following: 'It is easier for a camel to pass through the eye of a needle than …'	**'… for a rich man to enter heaven.'**
16	Name the twin sons of Isaac and Rebekah.	**Esau and Jacob**
17	How many times did Satan appear to Jesus in the wilderness?	**3 times**
18	Who could not speak until his son was born, because he did not believe the angel's word?	**Zacharias**
19	What was the Jewish high court called during Jesus' life time?	**Sanhedrin**
20	When Pharoah asked Moses and Aaron for a miracle, what happened?	**Aaron cast his rod down and it turned into a serpent**

LEVEL C

1	What language did Christ use during his life?	**Aramaic**
2	Name the prophet who was fed by ravens.	**Elijah**
3	What was the land of Tyre and Sidon also known as?	**Phoenicia**
4	Who was the chief priest who tried Jesus?	**Ciaphus**
5	What was the name of Moses' mother?	**Jochebed**
6	Name Enoch's son.	**Methuselah**
7	To whom did Jesus say, 'Because you have seen me you have believed'?	**Thomas**
8	What was the purpose of the Zealots?	**To drive the Romans from the land**
9	Name the stone monument that Samuel set up after a great victory over the Philistines.	**Ebenezer**
10	Name King Solomon's mother.	**Bathsheba**

Literature

LEVEL A

1 What was Aesop famous for? . . . . **His fables**

2 What type of novels did Barbara Cartland write? . . . . . **Romantic**

3 Who wrote *The Last of the Mohicans*? . . . . . . **James Fenimore Cooper**

4 Daniel Defoe wrote about a man shipwrecked on a desert island. Name the book. . . . . *Robinson Crusoe*

5 Kenneth Grahame wrote a book about a Toad, a Mole, a Badger and a Rat. What was the title? . . . . *The Wind in the Willows*

6 Whose travels did Jonathan Swift write about? . . . . . **Gulliver's**

7 Who wrote *Oliver Twist*, *Great Expectations*, *David Copperfield* and many more? . . . . **Charles Dickens**

8 Lewis Carroll wrote a book about dream adventures. What was it called? . . . . *Alice in Wonderland*

9 Every cub/scout reads a book by Rudyard Kipling about animals. What is it called? . . . . *Jungle Book*

10 Who was the secret agent created by Ian Fleming? . . . . **James Bond**

LEVEL B

1 An American author wrote a book about a great white whale that is hunted by Captain Ahab. What was the title? . . . . . *Moby Dick*

2 *For Whom the Bell Tolls* and *A Farewell to Arms* were written by whom? . . . . **Ernest Hemingway**

3 Who was the detective that Sir Conan Doyle wrote about? . . **Sherlock Holmes**

4 What is the title of the novel by Stephen Crane that tells the story of Henry Fleming's experiences during the American Civil War? . *The Red Badge of Courage*

5 Name the author of *Brideshead Revisited*. . . . . . . **Evelyn Waugh**

6 Who wrote *Sons and Lovers* and *The Virgin and the Gypsy*? . . **D H Lawrence**

7 Harriet Beecher Stowe wrote a famous book about slavery in the USA. What was the title? . . . . *Uncle Tom's Cabin*

8 Who was the heroine in *Wuthering Heights*? . . . . . . **Catherine**

9 John Wyndham wrote a book about plants taking over the world. What is the book called? . . . . ***The Day of the Triffids***

10 On which train does one of Agatha Christie's murders take place? **Orient Express**

11 In the Babar books, who did Babar the elephant marry? . . . **Celeste**

12 Who wrote *Animal Farm* and *Nineteen Eighty-Four*? . . . . **George Orwell**

13 On what subject does John le Carre base his novels? . . . **Spies and the secret service**

14 Where was Rudyard Kipling born? . . . . **Bombay**

15 Who wrote *The Old Wives' Tale*? . . . . **Arnold Bennett**

16 Whose autobiography was called *The Moon's a Balloon*? . **David Niven**

17 In which book does the phrase 'Fifteen men on a dead man's chest' play an important part? . . . . ***Treasure Island***

18 Where were the Joad family going in the novel by John Steinbeck titled *The Grapes of Wrath*? . . . . **California**

19 How many leagues under the sea did Jules Verne write about? . **20,000**

20 Who wrote *Pride and Prejudice*? . . . . **Jane Austen**

LEVEL C

1 What was Kingsley Amis' first novel? . . . . ***Lucky Jim***

2 In which book would you find the characters Ralph and Piggy? . ***Lord of the Flies***

3 Which famous Norwegian dramatist wrote about *A Doll's House*? **Henrik Ibsen**

4 Who wrote *The Three Sisters*, *The Cherry Orchard* and *The Seagull*? **Anton Chekov**

5 Name the author of *Breakheart Pass* . . . . **Alistair Maclean**

6 Who wrote *My Uncle Oswald*? . . . . **Roald Dahl**

7 In which play does Caliban appear? . . . . ***The Tempest***

8 In *The Pickwick Papers*, who was Mr Pickwick's cockney servant? **Sam Weller**

9 Who wrote *She Stoops to Conquer*? . . . . **Oliver Goldsmith**

10 Who created Frankenstein? . . . . **Mary Shelley**

The World Wars

LEVEL A

1	In which year did the First World War begin?	**1914**
2	Which particular race of people did Hitler persecute?	**Jews**
3	Of which country was Mussolini leader?	**Italy**
4	In which year was the Battle of Britain?	**1940**
5	What were German submarines called?	**U-boats**
6	What was Hitler's first name?	**Adolf**
7	What happened on 3 September 1939?	**The Second World War was declared**
8	Who worked in the factories when Britain was at war?	**Women**
9	What does RAF stand for?	**Royal Air Force**
10	What nationality was Mountbatten?	**British**

LEVEL B

1	What was the German Air Force called?	**Luftwaffe**
2	What were Utah, Omaha, Gold, Juno and Sword code names for in the Second World War?	**'D' Day landing beaches**
3	What were the Japanese suicide pilots called?	**Kamikaze**
4	What was the name of Hitler's master race?	**Aryan**
5	Where did every available boat in the South of England sail to rescue 338,000 troops?	**Dunkirk**
6	When was VE day?	**8 May 1945**
7	Which event brought the United States into the Second World War?	**Japanese attack on Pearl Harbor**
8	Who made the decision to drop an atomic bomb on Japan?	**Roosevelt**
9	Which American officer, later to become President, commanded PT109 in the Second World War?	**Lieutenant John F Kennedy**
10	The German invasion of which country on 1 September 1939 triggered off the Second World War?	**Poland**
11	What did the Germans call a tank division in the Second World War?	**Panzer**

12 Which general, refusing to surrender on the collapse of France, raised and led the Free French fighting forces? . . . . **General de Gaulle**

13 Where in the Western desert of North Africa was there a battle in 1942? . . . . **El Alamein**

14 What was the collective name for Britain, France, the USA and other friendly nations during the war? . . . . . . **Allies**

15 Who was Hitler's deputy who flew to Scotland in May 1941 with proposals for a compromise peace? . . . . **Rudolf Hess**

16 What does Reich mean? . . . . **Empire**

17 What does 'Führer' mean? . . . . **Leader**

18 In Operation Sealion, which country did Hitler propose to attack? **Britain**

19 Who announced 'Czechoslovakia has ceased to exist'? . . . **Hitler**

20 Who was the controller of Nazi propaganda during the Second World War? . . . . **Goebbels**

LEVEL C

1 Which agreement did Hitler violate by crossing the Czech border? **The Munich Agreement**

2 What was the German word meaning 'lightning war'? . . . **Blitzkrieg**

3 Name the three heads of state who met at the Yalta Conference? **Churchill, Stalin, Roosevelt**

4 Where was the document that formally concluded the Second World War signed? . . . . **Rheims, France**

5 Which treaty put forward by Woodrow Wilson in 1919 was based on 14 points? . . . . **Treaty of Versailles**

6 Which British statesman resigned after the German invasion of Holland, Belgium and Luxembourg in 1940? . . . . . . **Neville Chamberlain**

7 Who was known as The Desert Fox? . . . . **Erwin Rommel**

8 What, in Second World War parlance, was a UXB? . . . . **Unexploded bomb**

9 What did Josip Broz call himself? . . . . **Marshall Tito**

10 Who said 'How the great democracies triumphed and so were able to resume the follies which had so nearly cost them their life'? . **Winston Churchill**

LEVEL A

1 What nationality was Benjamin Britten? . . . . . . **British**
2 From what famous Oratorio by Handel does the *Halleluia Chorus* come? . . . . *Messiah*
3 Mendelssohn wrote some music about a cave. What was it? . *Fingel's Cave*
4 With what instrument do you associate Yehudi Menuhin? . . **Violin**
5 Mars, Venus, Saturn are movements of what suite by Gustav Holst? *Planet Suite*
6 Finish this title – *The Pirates of* . . . . *Penzance*
7 Who composed the music for the ballet *Swan Lake*? . . . . *Tchaikovsky*
8 How many musicians are there in a quartet? **4**
9 What name is given to the stick which the conductor uses to give directions to the orchestra? . . . . **Baton**
10 Who introduced the waltz? . . . . **Strauss**

LEVEL B

1 Who wrote the *Water Music*? . . . . **Handel**
2 How many notes are there in an octave? **8**
3 What is the name given to the deepest singing voice? . . . **Basso profundo**
4 How many strings has a violin? **4**
5 What is chamber music? . . . . **Music for small groups of instruments**
6 What does the musical term *forte* mean? . . . . **Loud or strong**
7 What is the name of the Gilbert and Sullivan operetta set in Japan? *The Mikado*
8 Who wrote the *Peer Gynt Suite*? . . . . **Grieg**
9 From what country does the opera singer Kiri Te Kanawa originate? . . . . **New Zealand**
10 What musical term is used to describe a male voice between tenor and bass? . . . . **Baritone**

11 What is a lyre? . . . . **Small harp**

12 With what instrument do you associate James Galway? . . . **Flute**

13 Who wrote the *William Tell Overture*? . . . . **Rossini**

14 What is opera bouffé? . . . . **Comic opera**

15 In an orchestra, which section do drums and tambourines belong to? . . . . **Percussion**

16 What is the highest female voice? . . . . **Soprano**

17 Who wrote the opera *La Boheme*? . . . . **Puccini**

18 From which work does the Can-can come? . . . . . . *Orpheus in the Underworld*

19 Name three stringed instruments . . . . **Violin, viola, cello, bass, guitar, mandolin and banjo**

20 What nationality was the composer Wagner? . . . . . **German**

LEVEL C

1 How many keys are there on a piano? **88**

2 Which sense did Beethoven lose? . . . . **His hearing**

3 Who wrote the opera *Madame Butterfly*? . . . . . . **Puccini**

4 Which instrument can play the highest note: the violin, the flute, the coronet or the xylophone? . . . . **The violin**

5 What does *pizzicato* mean? . . . . **Plucking of strings**

6 In which century did Chopin live? . . . . **The nineteenth**

7 Which instrument of the orchestra usually has 47 strings? . . **The harp**

8 Who wrote the *Moonlight Sonata*? . . . . **Beethoven**

9 With what instrument do you associate Paganini? . . . . **Violin**

10 How many lines in a stave? **5**

Abbreviations

LEVEL A

What do the following abbreviations stand for?

1 CD . . . . **Compact disc**
2 ETA . . . . **Estimated time of arrival**
3 BBC . . . . **British Broadcasting Corporation**
4 IQ . . . . **Intelligence Quotient**
5 VIP . . . . **Very Important Person**
6 UFO . . . . **Unidentified Flying Object**
7 AA . . . . **Alcoholics Anonymous/Automobile Association**
8 RIP . . . . **Rest in Peace**
9 HRH . . . . **Her (His) Royal Highness**
10 COD . . . . **Cash on Delivery**

LEVEL B

1 WHO . . . . **World Health Organization**
2 GMT . . . . **Greenwich Mean Time**
3 FBI . . . . **Federal Bureau of Investigation**
4 PS . . . . **Postscript**
5 MD . . . . **Doctor of Medicine**
6 AIDS . . . . **Acquired Immune Deficiency Syndrome**
7 RSVP . . . . **Répondez s'il vous plaît**
8 OBE . . . . **Officer of the Order of the British Empire**
9 CID . . . . **Criminal Investigation Department**
10 UN . . . . **United Nations**

11	VHF	. . . .	Very High Frequency
12	POW	. . . .	Prisoner of War
13	BC	. . . .	Before Christ
14	ID	. . . .	Identification
15	GI	. . . .	US armed forces serviceman
16	AD	. . . .	Anno Domini (In the year of our Lord)
17	NATO	. . . .	North Atlantic Treaty Organization
18	ESP	. . . .	Extra-Sensory Perception
19	MS	. . . .	Manuscript, Multiple Sclerosis
20	YMCA	. . . .	Young Men's Christian Association

LEVEL C

1	ISBN	. . . .	International Standard Book Number
2	NASA	. . . .	National Aeronautics and Space Administration
3	IOC	. . . .	International Olympics Committee
4	UDI	. . . .	Unilateral Declaration of Independence
5	SALT	. . . .	Strategic Arms Limitation Talks
6	IPA	. . . .	International Phonetic Alphabet
7	ITO	. . . .	International Trade Organization
8	GHQ	. . . .	General Headquarters
9	GATT	. . . .	General Agreement on Tariffs and Trade
10	AWOL	. . . .	Absent Without Official Leave

Parts of the Human Body

LEVEL A

1 Which protective cage surrounds the heart and lungs? . . . **Rib cage**
2 What is the watery secretion produced in the mouth called? . **Saliva**
3 What is produced in the ear to prevent dust from entering? . **Wax**
4 What is the heart's function? . . . . **To pump blood round the body**
5 What is the hinged bone of the mouth called? . . . . **Jaw**
6 Name the organ of smell. . . . . **Nose**
7 When you breathe in where does the air go? . . . . . **Into the lungs**
8 Where is the retina? . . . . **In the eye**
9 How many livers does each person have? **1**
10 When food is swallowed where does it go? . . . . . **Into the stomach**

LEVEL B

1 What does the cranium protect? . . . . **The brain**
2 What is the largest bone in the body? . . . . . **Femur**
3 Where is the sacrum? . . . . **Base of the spine**
4 Where is the thyroid gland? . . . . **Front of the neck**
5 What is the common name for the mammary glands? . . **Breasts**
6 Which organ has its blood supply from the coronary artery? . **Heart**
7 Where would you find plasma and platelets? . . . . **In the blood**
8 Where are the organs of balance found? . . . . . **In the ear**
9 What is found within the internal cavities of the bones? . . **Marrow**
10 Where is the jugular vein near the surface? . . . . . **In the neck**

11 What is the common name for the tibia? . . . . . . **Shin bone**

12 Where is the sciatic nerve? . . . . **Extends from the base of the spine down the leg**

13 What is the general difference between veins and arteries? . **Arteries carry blood from the heart to the body, veins return it to the heart**

14 Give the more common name of the vertebral column. . . . **Spine or backbone**

15 Where would you find carpals? . . . . **In the wrist**

16 Where are gastric juices produced? . . . . **In the stomach**

17 What is the common name for the patella? . . . . . **Knee cap**

18 What are the two large chambers of the heart? . . . . **Left and right ventricles**

19 Name the medical term for the gullet. . . . . . . **Oesophagus**

20 Name the medical term for the collar bone. . . . . . **Clavicle**

LEVEL C

1 Which artery enters the kidneys? . . . . **Renal**

2 How many vertebrae do we have? **33**

3 What type of joint is the hip? . . . . **Ball and socket**

4 What is the name of the fluid found in all joints? . . . . **Synovial fluid**

5 What does the lachrymal gland produce? . . . . . **Tears**

6 What is the name of the muscular sheet of tissue between the thorax and abdomen? . . . . **Diaphragm**

7 What are the digit bones called? . . . . **Phalanges**

8 Which gland produces insulin? . . . . **Pancreas**

9 After bile is produced in the liver, where is it stored? . . . **Gall bladder**

10 Which part of the tongue is sensitive to bitterness? . . . . **Back**

History

LEVEL A

1 Which King of England had six wives? . . . . . . **Henry VIII**
2 What political party did John F Kennedy represent? . . . . **The Democrats**
3 Which King of England was called the Lionheart? . . . . **Richard I**
4 In which year did the Second World War end? **1945**
5 Which ancient civilization built the Pyramids? . . . . . **Egyptians**
6 In which country did Buddhism originate? . . . . . **India**
7 Who travelled in the *Mayflower* to New England? . . . . **Pilgrim Fathers**
8 In which country was the Boer War fought? . . . . . **South Africa**
9 Who succeeded George VI on the British throne? . . . . **Queen Elizabeth II**
10 Who was the first man to land on the moon? . . . . . **Neil Armstrong**

LEVEL B

1 On what date did America declare its independence from Britain? **4 July 1776**
2 How many soldiers did a Roman centurion command? . . . **100**
3 Which Queen of England ruled for only 9 days? . . . . . **Lady Jane Grey**
4 What nationality was Hitler? . . . . **Austrian**
5 Which Prime Minister said, 'I have nothing to offer but blood, toil, tears and sweat'? . . . . **Winston Churchill**
6 Which Russian fortress, incorporating palaces and churches, became the seat of modern government? . . . . . . **The Kremlin**
7 Who succeeded Queen Victoria? . . . . **Edward VII**
8 Name the first president of the United States. . . . . **George Washington**
9 Which building in Rome was the arena where people were thrown to the lions? . . . . **The Colosseum**
10 Who was the first Prime Minister of the independent state of Israel? . . . . **David Ben-Gurion**

11	What destroyed Nagasaki in the Second World War?	**Atomic bomb**
12	When was the Great Fire of London?	**1666**
13	Which country was once known as Gaul?	**France**
14	What did Samuel Colt patent in 1835?	**The revolver**
15	Which Greek poet told the story of the Trojan war?	**Homer**
16	Who launched the Cultural Revolution in China?	**Mao Tse-tung**
17	What was the international crisis during John F Kennedy's presidency that took the world close to nuclear war?	**Cuban missile crisis**
18	Who founded the Fascist party in Italy in 1919?	**Mussolini**
19	In 1937 the Irish Free State changed its name to what?	**Eire**
20	How many times have the Olympic Games been cancelled due to war?	**3 – 1916, 1940 and 1944**

LEVEL C

1	The Caribbean and Pacific Ocean were linked by which canal in 1914?	**Panama Canal**
2	Who were the Hittites?	**A race which lived 4,000 years ago**
3	Lenin was the leading light of which revolutionary party in Russia?	**Bolsheviks**
4	Name the first king to reign over both England and Scotland?	**James I England, James VI Scotland**
5	When was the French Revolution?	**1789-99**
6	Into how many tribes were the Israelites divided?	**12**
7	What name was given to the operation to liberate Kuwait from Iraqi invaders?	**Operation Desert Storm**
8	When was the Suez Canal first opened?	**1869**
9	When was the Spanish Civil War?	**1936-39**
10	What was formally announced by George Bush and Mikhail Gorbachev on 3 December 1989?	**End of the Cold War**

Cookery

LEVEL A

1 What is brine? . . . . **Salt and water**
2 Which meat is served with mint sauce? . . . . . . **Lamb**
3 Which vegetables are 'petit pois'? . . . . **Peas**
4 Shallots and chives are types of what? . . . . . . **Onions**
5 Frogs legs and snails are delicacies in which European country? **France**
6 What liquid are onions pickled in? . . . . **Vinegar**
7 What does the term *par boiled* mean? . . . . . . **Partially cooked by boiling**
8 How do you make fresh cream thicken? . . . . . . **Whisk it**
9 Which meat is apple sauce served with? . . . . . . **Pork**
10 What is the main ingredient in an omelette? . . . . . **Egg**

LEVEL B

1 What are sweetbreads? . . . . **Glands of calves or lambs**
2 Why is steak sometimes beaten before cooking? . . . . **To tenderize it**
3 What is sorbet? . . . . **Water-ice made from fruit juice or puree**
4 Why don't strawberries freeze well? . . . . **Because of their high water content**
5 What is deer meat known as? . . . . **Venison**
6 Which kind of wine should be served chilled and which at room temperature? . . . . **White chilled, red at room temperature**
7 What is shortening? . . . . **Any fat for pastry making**
8 What does basting mean? . . . . **Ladling melted fat over roasted meat**
9 Which Italian cheese is traditionally served with spaghetti bolognaise? . . . . **Parmesan**
10 What is goulash? . . . . **Beef stew, usually with paprika**

11	What is the process of handling dough in bread-making called?	**Kneading**
12	What is a *poussin*?	**Baby chicken**
13	From which country does biryani originate?	**India**
14	What is the least nutritious fruit in the world?	**Cucumber**
15	What are the main ingredients of Paella?	**Rice and mixed seafood**
16	What is suet composed of?	**Fat that surrounds animal organs**
17	In an American restaurant, if you asked for a dish to be cooked *over easy* what would the dish be?	**Fried eggs**
18	What is the difference in nutritional value between a brown egg and a white egg?	**They are the same**
19	What do the Italians call their strong dark coffee served in small cups?	**Espresso**
20	What are croutons served with?	**Soups or salads**

LEVEL C

1	What is a vegetarian who eats dairy products known as?	**Lacto-vegetarian**
2	Which herb is used to flavour pickled cucumbers?	**Dill**
3	What name is given to a sort of thin pancake which is eaten throughout Mexico?	**Tortilla**
4	What is the name given to potatoes mashed, bound with egg, coated with breadcrumbs and fried in deep fat?	**Croquettes**
5	Which fruit has the highest protein value?	**Avocado pear**
6	What does *Lyonnaise* mean?	**With a garnish of fried onion**
7	What natural setting agent does a fruit need to make a good jam?	**Pectin**
8	What is a yam?	**Sweet potato**
9	What are the principal ingredients in mayonnaise?	**Egg yolk, oil and lemon juice or vinegar**
10	What is sauerkraut?	**A German dish of pickled cabbage**

LEVEL A

1 Complete the following: 'Christmas is coming, the goose is getting fat …' . . . . **'Please put a penny in the old man's hat'**

2 What was Wordsworth's first name? . . . . **William**

3 Who blew his pipe and charmed all the rats into following him? . **Pied Piper of Hamelin**

4 Complete the following: 'I had a little nut tree, nothing would it bear …' . . . . **'But a silver nutmeg and a golden pear'**

5 Who was the American poet and critic who wrote the book *Tales of Mystery and Imagination*? . . . . **Edgar Allan Poe**

6 Complete the following: 'Water water everywhere …' . . . **'Nor any drop to drink'**

7 What is an elegy? . . . . **A poem of lamentation, often for someone dead**

8 Who wrote *The Song of Hiawatha*? . . . . **Henry Wadsworth Longfellow**

9 Finish this line from Blake's poem: 'And did those feet in …' . **'Ancient times'**

10 According to the song, where is John Brown's body? . . . . **In the grave**

LEVEL B

1 Who wrote *The Rime of the Ancient Mariner*? . . . . . **Samuel Taylor Coleridge**

2 How many lines does a sonnet have? **14**

3 Who wrote a book of poems for children called *Old Possum's Book of Practical Cats*? . . . . **T S Eliot**

4 Complete the following: 'Kubla …' . . . . **'Khan'**

5 Who wrote *Canterbury Tales*? . . . . **Chaucer**

6 Who, commonly known for her poetry, wrote about her nervous breakdown in a novel called *The Bell Jar*? . . . . . . **Sylvia Plath**

7 What is a Poet Laureate? . . . . **Queen's poet, crowned with a laurel, honoured until death**

8 Which Victorian poet eloped with an invalid who was also a poet? **Robert Browning**

9 Who wrote *Paradise Lost*? . . . . **John Milton**

10 Which poet wrote *Ode to a Skylark* and *Ode to the West Wind*? . **Percy B Shelley**

11 What is blank verse? . . . . **Poetry which does not rhyme but has rhythm**

12 *Ulysses* was written by which famous poet? . . . . . **Alfred Lord Tennyson**

13 From which country does a haiku poem originate? . . . . **Japan**

14 'Half a league half a league half a league onwards'. Which famous poem does this come from? . . . . **The Charge of the Light Brigade**

15 Who was Hiawatha's father? . . . . **The West Wind (Mudjekeewis)**

16 Name Edward Lear's famous poem about an animal and a bird? . **The Owl and the Pussycat**

17 Who wrote the poem *If*? . . . . **Rudyard Kipling**

18 According to Shakespeare which quality is not strained? . . **Mercy. 'The quality of mercy is not strained'**

19 In the poem by Kipling, what was Gunga Din's job? . . . . **Water carrier**

20 The American poet Robert Frost won a prize for his poetry in 1924, 1931, 1937 and 1943. What was the prize? . . . . . **Pulitzer Prize for Poetry**

LEVEL C

1 Which talented poet wrote detective stories under the pseudonym Nicholas Blake? . . . . **C Day Lewis**

2 Who wrote the epic poems the *Iliad* and the *Odyssey*? . . . **Homer**

3 Who wrote the *Divine Comedy*? . . . . **Dante**

4 Which English novelist after writing *Jude the Obscure* wrote only poetry? . . . . **Thomas Hardy**

5 Who wrote *Don Juan*? . . . . **Lord Byron**

6 Name the author of *Lord of the Rings*. . . . . . . **J R R Tolkien**

7 Who wrote *Morte d'Arthur*? . . . . **Alfred Tennyson**

8 Name the American 19th-century poetess who was a recluse by the age of 30, dressing in white and carrying on friendships through correspondence? . . . . **Emily Dickinson**

9 What were Lord Byron's first names? . . . . **George Gordon**

10 What was hung around the neck of the Ancient Mariner? . . **The albatross**

LEVEL A

1 Of which country is the shamrock the national emblem? . . . **Ireland**
2 Which country do Danes come from? . . . . **Denmark**
3 Rotterdam is the chief port of which country? . . . . . **Netherlands (Holland)**
4 Which animal appears on the Welsh flag? . . . . . **Dragon**
5 Which winter sport is the main tourist attraction of the Alps? . **Skiing**
6 To which country do the islands of Majorca and Ibiza belong? . **Spain**
7 Which country did the Berlin Wall divide? . . . . . **Germany**
8 In which country does the canal city of Venice lie? . . . . **Italy**
9 What is the most famous French sparkling wine? . . . . **Champagne**
10 Where is Belfast? . . . . **Northern Ireland**

LEVEL B

1 In which country is Mount Etna? . . . . **Sicily**
2 Which sea port of the Isle of Wight is famous for its annual
sailing regatta? . . . . **Cowes**
3 Which European city is served by Schiphol Airport? . . . **Amsterdam**
4 Name Europe's foremost opera house situated in Milan. . . **La Scala**
5 Which principality is known for its casino at Monte Carlo? . . **Monaco**
6 What is the large wooded mountainous region in south-west
Germany called? . . . . **Black Forest**
7 Name the rocky promontory at the southern tip of Spain 3¾ miles
long and ¾ mile wide . . . . **Gibraltar**
8 Paris is situated on which river? . . . . **Seine**
9 What stretch of water separates Britain from France? . . . **English Channel**
10 Which country lies to the west of Spain? . . . . . . **Portugal**

11	Edelweiss is the national flower of which country?	**Austria**
12	What is the major river running through Germany and into Holland?	**Rhine**
13	Name the small country situated between France, Belgium and Germany.	**Luxembourg**
14	What is the large island in the Mediterranean belonging to France called?	**Corsica**
15	Which European country borders the Aegean Sea?	**Greece**
16	Which countries lie to the south of Poland?	**Czech Republic and Slovakia (formerly Czechoslovakia)**
17	Of which country is the peseta the currency?	**Spain**
18	What is the name of the area of rough seas between Northern Spain and France?	**Bay of Biscay**
19	Into which sea does the river Danube flow?	**Black Sea**
20	What is the mountain range between Spain and France called? .	**Pyrenees**

LEVEL C

1	What two countries does the Brenner Pass connect? . . .	**Italy and Austria**
2	Which river enters the North Sea at Hamburg?	**Elbe**
3	What currency is used in Portugal?	**Escudo**
4	On which island is the Valetta Carnival held?	**Malta**
5	Serbia and Macedonia are states found in which country? . .	**Yugoslavia**
6	What is Great Aletsch?	**A glacier in the Alps**
7	Which is the longest river in Britain?	**Severn**
8	What is the name of the famous ice cavern in Austria? . . .	**Dachstein**
9	Name the chief industrial town in Belgium	**Liege**
10	In which country is Magyar spoken?	**Hungary**

Geography: The Americas

LEVEL A

1 Which country in North America is the largest in area? . . . **Canada**
2 Which country in Latin America is the largest in area? . . . **Brazil**
3 Washington DC is the capital of which country? . . . . **USA**
4 What are the Rockies? . . . . **Chain of mountains in North America**
5 What is the famous long river which runs through the jungles of Latin America? . . . . **Amazon**
6 On which side of Latin America do the Andes Mountains run? . **West**
7 What is the main crop harvested in Canada? . . . . . **Wheat**
8 What is the most southernmost tip of Latin America called? . **Cape Horn**
9 What is the famous canal in Central America? . . . . **Panama**
10 Which country lies to the south of the USA? . . . . . **Mexico**

LEVEL B

1 What is the national emblem of Canada? . . . . . . **Maple leaf**
2 What twentieth-century manufacturing industry is centred in Detroit? . . . . **Car**
3 The highest lake in the world is on the border between Peru and Bolivia. Name it . . . . **Titicaca**
4 Which Latin American country is famous for its coffee export? . **Brazil**
5 What are the Mounties? . . . . **Royal Canadian Mounted Police**
6 In which bay is the island of Alcatraz? . . . . . . **San Francisco**
7 Which country lies to the west of Argentina? . . . . . **Chile**
8 Which is the largest island in the West Indies? . . . . **Cuba**
9 Name the Mormon world capital city. . . . . **Salt Lake City**
10 Which river runs within the Grand Canyon? . . . . . **Colorado River**

11	How many Great Lakes are there?	5
12	What stretch of water joins Lake Ontario with the Atlantic?	**St Lawrence River**
13	What language is chiefly spoken in the province of Quebec?	**French**
14	Where is Puerto Rico?	**Island in the Caribbean**
15	Which US city is known as 'the windy city'?	**Chicago**
16	In which country are the following cities – Rosario, Buenos Aires and Cordoba?	**Argentina**
17	New Orleans is near the estuary of which river?	**Mississippi**
18	In which state of the USA is Los Angeles?	**California**
19	In which state of the USA is Miami?	**Florida**
20	What are the group of states in the far north east of the USA called?	**New England**

LEVEL C

1	What is the chief mineral mined in Bolivia?	**Tin**
2	Where would you find the Bronx?	**New York**
3	Name two of the Prairie Provinces	**Manitoba, Alberta, Saskatchewan**
4	Which country owns Greenland?	**Denmark**
5	Which city is known as 'the mile-high city'?	**Denver**
6	What is a Hawaiian garland known as?	**Lei**
7	Which country lies between Panama and Nicaragua?	**Costa Rica**
8	What part of Canada bordering Alaska was the scene of the great gold rush?	**Yukon**
9	Brasilia was built to reduce the population of which city?	**Rio de Janeiro**
10	In which state in the USA is Milwaukee?	**Wisconsin**

Geography: Rest of World

LEVEL A

1 Which country lies south east of Australia? . . . . . . **New Zealand**
2 Which country has the largest population in the world? . . . **China**
3 What is the largest desert in North Africa called? . . . . **Sahara**
4 Which is the highest mountain in the world? . . . . . . **Everest**
5 With which country do you associate the following: sheep farming, boomerangs and *Waltzing Matilda*? . . . . **Australia**
6 Which is the largest country in the world? . . . . . **Russian Federation**
7 What is the name of the ocean between Europe and America? . **Atlantic**
8 What is the southernmost country in Africa called? . . . **South Africa**
9 What precious metal is mined in Johannesburg, South Africa? . **Gold**
10 What line divides the Northern and Southern Hemispheres? . **Equator**

LEVEL B

1 What was the previous name for Sri Lanka? . . . . . . **Ceylon**
2 From which country do the Aborigines come? . . . . . **Australia**
3 Where is the Bering Sea? . . . . **Between Russia and Alaska**
4 Name the people that live in the Congo Forest who are the smallest people in the world . . . . **Pygmies**
5 What is the most important crop grown in the Monsoon lands? . **Rice**
6 What currency is used in India? . . . . **Rupee**
7 In which country is Mecca? . . . . **Saudi Arabia**
8 In which country are Kuala Lumpur and Penang? . . . . **Malaysia**
9 What canal joins the Mediterranean and Red Seas? . . . . **Suez**
10 Which river divides Zambia and Zimbabwe? . . . . . . **Zambezi**

11 In which country would you find Nairobi and Mombasa? . . . **Kenya**

12 Which country lies south of the Straits of Gibraltar? . . . . **Morocco**

13 Which country lies to the east of the Red Sea? . . . . . **Saudi Arabia**

14 In which country would you find the two rivers Indus and Ganges? **India**

15 Where is Hiroshima? . . . . **Japan**

16 Name the highest mountain in the Alps. . . . . . . **Mont Blanc**

17 Europe is separated from Asia by which mountain range? . . **Urals**

18 Which country lies between Afghanistan and India? . . . . **Pakistan**

19 What is the main export from Sri Lanka? . . . . . . **Tea**

20 Where is the Gobi Desert? . . . . **China and Mongolia**

LEVEL C

1 What is the large South African desert which lies mainly in
Botswana called? . . . . **Kalahari**

2 Which sea lies west of New Zealand? . . . . **Tasman Sea**

3 In which country is Kilimanjaro? . . . . **Tanzania**

4 Name two of the countries which border Ethiopia. . . . . **Sudan, Kenya, Somalia**

5 Where would you find Table Mountain? . . . . **Cape Town**

6 Where is the Gulf of Carpentaria? . . . . **Northern Australia**

7 Where would you find Mount Cook? . . . . **South Island, New Zealand**

8 Which sea lies to the north of Iran? . . . . **Caspian**

9 What does UAE stand for? . . . . **United Arab Emirates**

10 Name the chief port of China . . . . **Shanghai**

LEVEL A

1 What is the name of the place where fruit trees like apples, pears and plums grow? . . . . **Orchard**

2 Which day is St Valentine's Day? . . . . **14 February**

3 What was the name given to a water filled ditch that surrounded a castle as a means of defence? . . . . **Moat**

4 If you were born at the end of May, which sign of the zodiac would you belong to? . . . . **Gemini**

5 If you sit on a horse without a saddle how are you said to ride? . **Bareback**

6 What would you make in a samovar? . . . . **Tea**

7 Which river does London stand on? . . . . **Thames**

8 How many points are there to the compass? **32**

9 How many days are there in January? **31**

10 Who wrote the play *A Midsummer Night's Dream*? . . . . **Shakespeare**

LEVEL B

1 What diffusion of rays from nuclear material causes serious illness? . . . . **Radiation**

2 Which oriental bean can be processed to make a meat substitute? **Soya**

3 Which is the world's smallest continent? . . . . . . **Australia**

4 Which famous woman was born on 21 April 1926? . . . . **Queen Elizabeth II**

5 What nationality was Hans Christian Anderson? . . . . . **Danish**

6 What is the name of the period of fasting from Ash Wednesday to Easter? . . . . **Lent**

7 Who wrote *Lady Chatterley's Lover*? . . . . **D H Lawrence**

8 In which US state is Fort Knox? . . . . **Kentucky**

9 What are pieces of meat on a skewer called? . . . . . **Kebab**

10 Which cavalry officer was killed at the battle of Little Big Horn? . **General Custer**

11	What is boiling point on the Fahrenheit scale?	**212 degrees**
12	What is deadly nightshade otherwise known as?	**Belladonna**
13	Of all books ever published which has sold the most copies? .	***The Bible***
14	What is the correct name for a guardsman's busby?	**Bearskin**
15	What does NCO stand for?	**Non-Commissioned Officer**
16	Which King of England had to hide in an oak tree to avoid capture by the Roundheads?	**Charles II**
17	The Egyptian Empire came to an end with the death of which queen?	**Cleopatra**
18	What are animals called that can live either on sea or land? . .	**Amphibians**
19	What do Welshmen wear in their lapels on St David's Day? . .	**Daffodils**
20	What is marijuana otherwise known as?	**Pot, grass**

LEVEL C

1	How did Mussolini die?	**He was shot while trying to escape to Switzerland**
2	What happened to Alaska on 29 March 1867?	**It was sold to the USA by Russia**
3	Name the negative electrode of an electrolytic cell	**Cathode**
4	In which country is Dominion day celebrated?	**Canada**
5	What was the 'tocsin bell'?	**A bell rung in times of danger**
6	Where were the Olympic Games held in 1968?	**Mexico City**
7	How many sides has a dodecahedron?	**12**
8	How many labours was Hercules called upon to perform? . .	**12**
9	What is the name given to coypu fur?	**Nutria**
10	Who was the Sun King?	**Louis XIV of France**

LEVEL A

1 What are mounds formed by windblown sand called? . . . **Dunes**
2 In which film is the song *Somewhere over the Rainbow* sung? . **The Wizard of Oz**
3 Which birth sign is represented by a lion? . . . . . **Leo**
4 Which tree produces acorns? . . . . **Oak**
5 Where is the poison in deadly snakes? . . . . . **In their fangs**
6 Where are you most likely to find a dragonfly? . . . . **Near water**
7 Who was Princess Anne's first husband? . . . . . **Captain Mark Phillips**
8 From which direction did the Wise Men come? . . . . **East**
9 What do you call a horse's fastest pace? . . . . . **Gallop**
10 What is a stickleback? . . . . **Fish**

LEVEL B

1 What is a pessimist? . . . . **Someone who expects the worst**
2 What is the right-hand side of a ship called? . . . . **Starboard**
3 What is the name of the secret American racist group which grew up during the Civil War? . . . . **Ku Klux Klan**
4 Which type of fat can increase the cholestrol level in blood? . . **Saturated fat**
5 In which year were silver coins made in cupronickel in Britain? . **1946**
6 Name the British sovereign's personal flag? . . . . . **The Royal Standard**
7 What is measured by a chronometer? . . . . . **Time**
8 Which language do most people in Mexico speak? . . . **Spanish**
9 Which bluish-white metal is used in galvanizing? . . . **Zinc**
10 What is a typhoon? . . . . **A destructive whirlwind**

11 What is the counting of a population known as? . . . . . **Census**

12 What colour does copper turn a flame? . . . . . . **Green**

13 Which monk had a great deal of power over the Russian royal family? . . . . **Rasputin**

14 What is dry ice? . . . . **Solid carbon dioxide**

15 If no matter which direction you walk you are going south, where are you? . . . . **North Pole**

16 What was a diplodocus? . . . . **Dinosaur**

17 What country lies between China and Russia? . . . . **Mongolia**

18 What colour robes do buddhist monks wear? . . . . **Saffron (yellow)**

19 What type of root does a crocus have? . . . . . . **Bulb**

20 In which country did the ancient Aztecs live? . . . . . **Mexico**

LEVEL C

1 Of what country was Alexander the Great ruler? . . . . . **Macedonia**

2 What is the name given to a line on a map joining places of the same barometric pressure? . . . . **Isobar**

3 Who discovered nuclear fusion in the early twentieth century? . **Rutherford**

4 What is a col? . . . . **A mountain pass**

5 Who was Capability Brown? . . . . **A famous eighteenth-century landscape gardener**

6 What were the citizens of ancient Greece renowned for their hardness and self-discipline called? . . . . **Spartans**

7 Who was the central male character of *Wuthering Heights*? . . **Heathcliff**

8 Which British newspaper was the first to publish a crossword? . ***Sunday Express***

9 What does an entomologist study? . . . . **Insects**

10 What is the F-15 Eagle? . . . . **Supersonic jet fighter**

LEVEL A

1	What are pinking shears?	**Dressmaking scissors with serrated blades**
2	What does the slang term *nosh* mean?	**Food**
3	What are the small boats that pull ships into harbours called?	**Tugs**
4	What do seals eat?	**Fish**
5	Which type of clover is said to be lucky?	**4-leafed**
6	Which Liverpool group sprang to fame with songs like *She Loves You* and *Please Please Me*?	**The Beatles**
7	What type of meat do you get from a cow?	**Beef**
8	Which animal has black and white stripes?	**Zebra**
9	When would you use a thimble?	**Sewing**
10	Who would wear a sari?	**Indian woman**

LEVEL B

1	What are animals called whose first food is their mother's milk?	**Mammals**
2	In which country is the Winter Palace?	**Russian Federation**
3	Which island is known as the Emerald Isle?	**Ireland**
4	Where is the Bridge of Sighs?	**Venice**
5	What is the English translation of *ad lib*?	**Off the cuff**
6	What does the expression 'to call a spade a spade' mean?	**Speak out plainly**
7	Who wrote *The Time Machine*?	**H G Wells**
8	What happened on 22nd November 1963?	**J F Kennedy was assassinated**
9	In the proverb, what killed the cat?	**Curiosity**
10	Who was the star of the Pink Panther series of films?	**Peter Sellers**

11	What is the name for someone who makes a study of birds?	**Ornithologist**
12	What is a prime number?	**One divisble only by itself or one**
13	What is the name of the cord that attaches a baby to its mother in the womb?	**Umbilical cord**
14	Name the longest snake in the world	**Python**
15	From which fish is caviare a product?	**Sturgeon**
16	Which insect passes on malaria?	**Mosquito**
17	What does the musical term *adagio* mean?	**Very slow**
18	Why do owls have to turn their heads right round when they want to look at something?	**Their eyeballs cannot move**
19	How many degrees are there in a circle?	**360**
20	Name the colours in the French flag?	**Blue, white and red**

LEVEL C

1	What was Joseph Vissarionovich Djugashvili better known as?	**Stalin**
2	What are salmon's eggs that hatch called?	**Alevins**
3	Who said 'He who can does. He who cannot teaches'? . . .	**George Bernard Shaw**
4	In which county in Scotland is Glasgow?	**Lanark**
5	What is Zephyr?	**The west wind**
6	Which country is the world's main exporter of tin?	**Malaysia**
7	In some flowers the nectary produces nectar. What do the anthers produce?	**Pollen**
8	What is Arthur's Seat?	**The highest of the 7 hills of Edinburgh, Scotland**
9	Which country has the most earthquakes?	**Japan**
10	Name the Welsh annual festival of the arts?	**Eisteddfod**

LEVEL A

1	What kind of doctor looks after animals' health?	**Veterinary surgeon**
2	What is a plume?	**Feather**
3	What kind of turf is cut for fuel?	**Peat**
4	Name the lines of latitude called the tropics.	**Cancer, Capricorn**
5	Name five colours of the rainbow.	**Red, orange, yellow, green, blue, indigo, violet**
6	Name the capital of Wales.	**Cardiff**
7	What is the name of the line passing round the centre of the Earth?	**Equator**
8	What is the marine tortoise called?	**Turtles**
9	What does a tailor make?	**Clothes**
10	Name three dairy products.	**Milk, cream, cheese, butter, yogurt**

LEVEL B

1	What is Fujiyama?	**A mountain in Japan**
2	In chess, what is another name for a castle?	**Rook**
3	What is an inscription on a tombstone called?	**An epitaph**
4	How many fluid ounces are there in a pint?	**20**
5	Which Russian Czar was known as 'the terrible'?	**Ivan**
6	What is the helmsman of a rowing boat called?	**Cox**
7	What are hieroglyphics?	**Symbols used in ancient writing**
8	Constantinople is the old name of which city?	**Istanbul**
9	What is the name for a Chinese ship?	**Junk**
10	What is the name for a person who makes hats?	**Milliner**

11	Which is the longest river in the world?	**Nile**
12	What can you do if you are bilingual?	**Speak two languages (fluently)**
13	In which country did paper originate?	**China**
14	What is measured in reams?	**Paper**
15	How many sides does a hexagon have?	**6**
16	What does C of S stand for?	**Church of Scotland**
17	What do you call a place in the desert where there is water?	**Oasis**
18	What are cacao beans used for?	**To make chocolate**
19	What colour is the German flag?	**Black, red and yellow**
20	From what plant is linen made?	**Flax**

LEVEL C

1	Who was Queen Elizabeth I's chief adviser?	**William Cecil**
2	What is the highest officer of a regiment called?	**Colonel**
3	Who wrote the novel *Gone With the Wind*?	**Margaret Mitchell**
4	What is the name of the willow whose pliable twigs are used in basket weaving?	**Osier**
5	Which opera by Verdi was written to celebrate the opening of the Suez Canal?	**Aida**
6	What pungent gas is strongly associated with smelling salts?	**Ammonia**
7	What is a Dicentra?	**Flower**
8	Where would you find the Liebritz mountains?	**On the moon**
9	Name the sea that lies between Greece and Asia Minor.	**Aegean**
10	Which book of the Old Testament follows Nehemiah?	**Esther**

LEVEL A

1 What is a siesta? . . . . **A short rest or nap**
2 What colour is an emerald? . . . . **Green**
3 What is another popular name for the badger? . . . . . **Brock**
4 Which bird can hold up to three gallons of water in a pouch below its beak? . . . . **Pelican**
5 The first day of which month is All Fools' Day? . . . . . **April**
6 Which wall is about 1,500 miles long? . . . . **Great Wall of China**
7 What is the name for a lake in Scotland? . . . . **Loch**
8 What precious stone could be found inside an oyster? . . . **Pearl**
9 From which country do koala bears come? . . . . . . **Australia**
10 How many legs does an insect have? **6**

LEVEL B

1 For what would you use an abacus? . . . . **Counting, calculating**
2 On which date is St Patrick's Day? . . . . **17 March**
3 Which day is St Andrew's Day? . . . . **30 November**
4 From what is ivory obtained? . . . . **Elephant tusks**
5 What is measured on the Richter Scale? . . . . . . **Earthquakes**
6 Which nerves supply the eyes? . . . . **Optic**
7 Which well known Israeli leader wore an eye patch? . . . . **Moshe Dayan**
8 How many circles are there on the Olympic flag? **5**
9 To what family of birds do lovebirds belong? . . . . . **Parrots**
10 What did the *Titanic* hit? . . . . **Iceberg**

11 In which country did the Olympic Games begin in 1896? . . . **Greece**

12 What is a rajah's wife called? . . . . **Ranee**

13 What is a long series of fast beats on a drum called? . . . **Roll**

14 Name an airport in Paris. . . . . **Orly, Charles de Gaulle**

15 Which sign of the zodiac is represented by the goat? . . . **Capricorn**

16 What is the name of the round heavy object attached to a chain which is thrown in athletics? . . . . **Hammer**

17 What is a tree-lined road called? . . . . **Avenue**

18 Who was the first black tennis player to win Wimbledon? . . **Arthur Ashe**

19 Who wrote *The Grapes of Wrath*? . . . . **John Steinbeck**

20 What is the outermost layer of the earth called? . . . . **The crust**

LEVEL C

1 Which English King founded Eton College? . . . . . **Henry VI**

2 What is the medical speciality concerned with illness in children called? . . . . **Paediatrics**

3 Which country's flag is white with a red disc? . . . . **Japan**

4 Who assassinated Abraham Lincoln? . . . . **John Wilkes Booth**

5 When was the Post Office tower in London built? . . . **1965**

6 What is the Icelandic parliament called? . . . . . . **Althing**

7 In Shakespeare's play, who killed Macbeth? . . . . . **Macduff**

8 Who lived in Haworth Parsonage? . . . . **The Brontë family**

9 What year was the Battle of Trafalgar? **1805**

10 What does a pantomimist neglect? . . . . **Speech**

LEVEL A

1 What relation is your brother's daughter to you? . . . . . **Niece**
2 What is dried grass used as animal fodder called? . . . . **Hay**
3 Which colour traditionally denotes danger? . . . . . **Red**
4 What is the sport of shooting with a bow called? . . . . **Archery**
5 If you are in your birthday suit what are you wearing? . . . **Nothing**
6 What did Dorothy in *The Wizard of Oz* wear on her feet? . . **Red shoes (Ruby slippers)**
7 Complete the following: Tom, Dick and . . . . . . **Harry**
8 What grows in a vineyard? . . . . **Grapes**
9 What is a locust? . . . . **A large grasshopper**
10 What do leeches suck? . . . . **Blood**

LEVEL B

1 How many carats does pure gold have? **24**
2 Who was Eva Braun? . . . . **Hitler's mistress**
3 Which fictional character lived in Baker Street? . . . . **Sherlock Holmes**
4 Who founded the first US detective agency in 1850? . . . **Allan Pinkerton**
5 On which US tycoon's life was the film *Citizen Kane* based? . **William Randolph Hearst**
6 A person who steals cattle is known as what? . . . . . **Rustler**
7 What have the following in common – Mussolini, Hitler and Franco? **All dictators**
8 What is the Star of Sierra Leone? . . . . **A rough uncut diamond**
9 Who was Moses' brother? . . . . **Aaron**
10 From what is *Pâté de foie gras* made? . . . . . . **Goose liver**

11 In which year did the *Titanic* sink? 1912
12 Which author created the character 'Peter Pan'? . . . . . J M Barrie
13 What is a ship's kitchen called? . . . . Galley
14 What is the name for a person who examines rock samples? . Geologist or mineralogist
15 Of which element is diamond a form? . . . . . . Carbon
16 What alcoholic drink do the Japanese make from rice? . . . Sake
17 What is one of the heaviest metals that is also pliable? . . . Lead
18 Which famous war was fought between 1854-56? . . . . Crimean War
19 Who started the first London police force? . . . . . . Sir Robert Peel
20 Who was the man who made Russia a Communist country? . . Lenin

LEVEL C

1 Who was the first woman to receive the Order of Merit in 1907? . Florence Nightingale
2 What is a bummaree? . . . . A market porter
3 What is the name given to a coral reef shaped like a ring or
   horseshoe round a lagoon? . . . . Atoll
4 Which volcano exploded in 1883? . . . . Mount Krakatoa
5 Who wrote a play called *The Circle*? . . . . Somerset Maugham
6 Boadicea was the queen of which tribe? . . . . . . Iceni
7 Who discovered penicillin? . . . . Alexander Fleming
8 What is nyctophobia a fear of? . . . . The dark
9 Who wrote the following line: 'Don't put your daughter on the
   stage Mrs Worthington'? . . . . Noel Coward
10 Which US president's desk bore the legend 'the buck stops here'? Harry S Truman

LEVEL A

1. Which vehicle is traditionally the home of gypsies? . . . . . **Caravan**
2. Which Tuesday is pancake day? . . . . **Shrove Tuesday**
3. To which animal family do the lion and domestic tabby belong? . **Cat**
4. What is the name of the rotating part of a windmill? . . . . **Sail**
5. Where is your funny bone? . . . . **Elbow**
6. Which sci-fi author wrote the screenplay for *2001: A Space Odyssey*? . . . . **Arthur C Clarke**
7. How many days in April? **30**
8. What does 'to mime' mean? . . . . **To act without speaking**
9. Where does solar energy come from? . . . . . . **The sun**
10. For what did Johann Sebastian Bach gain fame? . . . . **Composing music**

LEVEL B

1. What is the day after Hallowe'en called? . . . . . . **All Saints' Day**
2. Which river does Berwick stand on? . . . . **Tweed**
3. What type of wine is described as *sec*? . . . . . . **Dry**
4. What is a torso? . . . . **Trunk of the human body**
5. Who was the commander of Apollo 11? . . . . . . **Neil Armstrong**
6. What is the crime of burning property called? . . . . **Arson**
7. What is the leader of the Church of Scotland called? . . . . **Moderator**
8. What is a Peruvian lion? . . . . **Puma**
9. Who or what is Lucifer? . . . . **Satan**
10. How are outlaws Parker and Barrow better known? . . . . **Bonnie and Clyde**

11	What type of gas comes from the North Sea?	**Natural**
12	What is the opening of a sweat gland called?	**Pore**
13	Where in London would you find the Royal Artillery Memorial? .	**Hyde Park Corner**
14	What is a dried plum called?	**Prune**
15	What is an impervious rock?	**One that will not let water pass through it**
16	What is a person who stuffs animals called?	**Taxidermist**
17	What are the long, narrow boats used on the canals of Venice called?	**Gondolas**
18	Where is the home of the Bolshoi Ballet?	**Bolshoi Theatre, Moscow**
19	When would a monk go to the religious service of vespers? . .	**In the evening**
20	'What goes up must come down'. What is this law called? . .	**Gravity**

LEVEL C

1	Pewter is an alloy of which metals?	**Tin and lead**
2	Who composed the *Carnival of Animals*?	**Saint-Saens**
3	Which branch of learning is named from the Greek for 'love of wisdom'?	**Philosophy**
4	What is the name of the tower in which Big Ben is housed? .	**St Stephen's Tower**
5	Which Roman Emperor is said to have played the fiddle while the city burned?	**Nero**
6	Which instrument was played by Orpheus?	**Lute**
7	Who wrote the novel *Moby Dick* in 1851?	**Herman Melville**
8	Which novel by Boris Pasternak was refused publication in the USSR?	***Doctor Zhivago***
9	Which substance is the main constituent of mothballs? . . .	**Camphor**
10	What is herpetology?	**Study of reptiles**

LEVEL A

1	Which insect is red with black spots?	**Ladybird**
2	In dice, what are 'snake eyes'?	**2**
3	What jumped over the moon in the nursery rhyme?	**Cow**
4	What is a dahlia?	**Flower**
5	What is frozen water called?	**Ice**
6	Which snake makes a noise by shaking its tail?	**Rattlesnake**
7	What is an apple seed called?	**Pip**
8	From which country does Haggis come?	**Scotland**
9	How many children has Queen Elizabeth II?	**4**
10	What is a baboon?	**A large monkey**

LEVEL B

1	What is the eye of a camera called?	**Lens**
2	What is the first day of Lent called?	**Ash Wednesday**
3	Which famous Russian male ballet dancer defected in 1961?	**Nureyev**
4	What nationality was Christopher Columbus?	**Italian**
5	Where did Davy Crockett die?	**The Alamo**
6	What is the name for a person who draws maps?	**Cartographer**
7	Who was King Arthur's magician?	**Merlin**
8	What are *homo sapiens*?	**Human beings**
9	Which is the fastest stroke in swimming?	**Crawl**
10	How many years does a silver wedding anniversary celebrate?	**25**

11 What is acrophobia? . . . . **Fear of heights**

12 What is a large bird's claw called? . . . . **Talon**

13 What is the animal that has a drooping moustache and tusks and is related to the seal? . . . . **Walrus**

14 What fruit is used to make the drink perry? . . . . . . **Pear**

15 What do copper and zinc make? . . . . **Brass**

16 Where would you find a delta? . . . . **At the mouth of a river**

17 What is a solo song in opera called? . . . . **Aria**

18 What is a bicycle for two riders called? . . . . **Tandem**

19 Ernest Hemingway wrote *A Farewell to* what? . . . . . **Arms**

20 For what is Waterford, Ireland, well known? . . . . . . **Crystal**

LEVEL C

1 What is the lithosphere? . . . . **The outer layer of the Earth's crust**

2 What are trichologists concerned with? . . . . **Hair**

3 What instrument represents the duck in *Peter and the Wolf*? . **Oboe**

4 Who was the Roman god of wine? . . . . **Bacchus**

5 What is a dewlap? . . . . **Flap of loose skin that hangs from the throat of an animal such as bloodhound or cow**

6 Name Britain's oldest university. . . . . **Oxford**

7 Who or what killed Cleopatra? . . . . **An asp**

8 To which bird family do the moorhen, coot and crane belong? . **Rail**

9 Which old testament book comes between *Joshua* and *Ruth*? . ***Judges***

10 Where would you find the grave of Karl Marx? . . . . . **Highgate Cemetary, London**

LEVEL A

1	What is the Sunday before Easter called?	**Palm Sunday**
2	Who is the patron saint of travellers?	**St Christopher**
3	What kind of place is the Sahara?	**Desert**
4	What is a young duck called?	**Duckling**
5	What is a matador?	**Bull fighter**
6	What is a thick mist called?	**Fog**
7	What is cured pig meat known as?	**Bacon**
8	What colour is jet?	**Black**
9	Complete the following: 'As light as a …'	**Feather**
10	What fruit is used to make cider?	**Apples**

LEVEL B

1	What is the word for a dread of confined places?	**Claustrophobia**
2	What was the robe worn by Roman citizens called?	**Toga**
3	What is the plural of fungus?	**Fungi**
4	In gardening, what is a savoy?	**Type of cabbage**
5	What is the last word in the Bible?	**Amen**
6	In which country was Alcoholics Anonymous set up in 1934?	**USA**
7	Which race of people speak yiddish?	**Jews**
8	Which camel has two humps?	**Bactrian**
9	Which is the name of a triangle in which two of the sides are equal in length?	**Isosceles**
10	Which animal has a bill like that of a duck?	**Platypus**

11	Who was the first known Norman King?	**William the Conqueror**
12	What is an aperitif?	**Pre-dinner drink**
13	Which zodiac sign is represented by scales?	**Libra**
14	What is a Molotov cocktail?	**A homemade bomb**
15	Name the planet furthest from the sun in our solar system.	**Pluto**
16	What does a rheostat control?	**Electric current**
17	Name the first letter of the Greek alphabet?	**Alpha**
18	What is the currency of Italy?	**Lira**
19	What was the first mass produced car?	**Model T Ford called** *Tin Lizzie*
20	Where are the headquarters of the United Nations?	**New York**

LEVEL C

1	In which country is the schilling a monetary unit?	**Austria**
2	In which London church is the Duke of Wellington buried?	**St Paul's Cathedral**
3	What is the stirrup-shaped bone of the ear called?	**Stapes**
4	Whom did William Shakespeare marry?	**Anne Hathaway**
5	What was the name of the hunchback of Notre-Dame?	**Quasimodo**
6	What is Tokay?	**Hungarian wine**
7	What is the Moslem fasting period called?	**Ramadan**
8	Who was the eldest son of Adam and Eve?	**Cain**
9	What does Golgotha, the name of the crucifixion, mean?	**Skull**
10	What is the calendar that we use today called?	**Gregorian calendar**

LEVEL A

1	Who was Robin Hood's fat friend?	**Friar Tuck**
2	What is a flat round soft cap, often worn by Frenchmen called?	**Beret**
3	What are cowboy films called?	**Westerns**
4	What is salami?	**Type of sausage**
5	How many days is 72 hours?	**3**
6	In which season do apples ripen?	**Autumn**
7	Where would you find antlers?	**On an animal's head**
8	Who was the fairy in *Peter Pan*?	**Tinker Bell**
9	Who wrote the novel *Treasure Island*?	**R L Stevenson**
10	What colour is a sapphire?	**Blue**

LEVEL B

1	Which Biblical book mentions 'A land flowing with milk and honey'?	**Exodus**
2	On which tree are catkins found?	**Hazel**
3	What is amnesia?	**Loss of memory**
4	Whose famous school days were spent at Rugby School?	**Tom Brown's**
5	What is the upright of a step called?	**Rise**
6	On which river is Vienna sited?	**Danube**
7	What does the Latin term *sub judice* mean?	**Under consideration**
8	What is seismology?	**Study of earthquakes**
9	On which island was Napoleon first exiled?	**Elba**
10	What are the women's quarters in a Mohammedan house called?	**Harem**

11 Name the international language. . . . . **Esperanto**

12 What sort of fruit is a morello? . . . . **Cherry**

13 Which country presented the USA with the Statue of Liberty? . **France**

14 Who attends to ailments of the feet? . . . . **Chiropodist**

15 Who was Spandau's last prisoner? . . . . **Rudolf Hess**

16 What is hydrophobia? . . . . **Fear of water**

17 What is an eye glass for one eye called? . . . . . . **Monocle**

18 Where was Cary Grant born? . . . . **Bristol**

19 What substance is burned to give out fragrant fumes during
    religious ceremonies? . . . . **Incense**

20 What were the ancient Egyptian kings called? . . . . . **Pharoahs**

LEVEL C

1 Which of Cole Porter's musicals was based on *The Taming of the
   Shrew*? . . . . *Kiss Me Kate*

2 Which point is opposite to the zenith? . . . . **Nadir**

3 What fine brown pigment is derived from the ink sac of the
   cuttlefish? . . . . **Sepia**

4 What find enabled man to read the writing that the Egyptians
   left behind? . . . . **Rosetta Stone**

5 Which family lived at *The Mill on the Floss*? . . . . . . **Tulliver**

6 With which cathedral is St Swithin connected? . . . . . **Winchester**

7 Who was the leader of the Hungarian revolt of 1956? . . . **Nagy**

8 In which year was the Sydney Opera House opened? . . . **1973**

9 When did Columbus sail to America? **1492**

10 Name the planet nearest the sun. . . . . **Mercury**

Also Available from Speechmark...

Speechmark publishes and distributes a wide range of creative resources providing exciting and appealing ideas for countless group activities. Listed below are just a few of these products – a full catalogue is available on request.

The Activity & Reminiscence Handbook
Hundreds of Ideas in 52 Weekly Sessions
Danny Walsh

This week-by-week guide provides a bumper book of original resource material for reminiscence and activities with older people for a whole year! Containing 52 selections of ideas and resource materials for each week of this year, this is an invaluable and easy to use resource relevant for both groups and individuals.

Creative Themes for Groupwork and Personal Development
Susan Pinn-Atkinson & Jenny Woolloff

Based around 30 themes, this practical resource provides flexible and adaptable ideas for groupwork sessions. The themes can be adapted and developed to match the exact needs and interests of the participants.

The Art Activity Manual
A Groupwork Resource
Marylyn Cropley

A simple, flexible and practical approach to art activities, this book enables group members to explore and discover their own level of artistic skills, creative styles and preferences and enables facilitators to find a fast, efficient and cost-effective way of meeting individual needs within an art group setting.

Games for Talking
Games for Talking is a unique series of boxed cards designed for speech & language therapists, occupational therapists, teachers and all group leaders. The three games can be used as icebreakers, warm-ups, as a stand-alone activity, or time fillers.

Let's Talk!
A very popular set of discussion and prompt cards designed for use by all groups.

Let's Mime!
A simple non-competitive charades game for groups of two or more people of any age.

Top 5
Another popular set of cards for conversation, group openers or for use simply as a fun game. Each card suggests a category for top five discussions.

For further information please contact

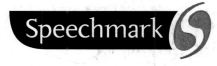

www.speechmark.net